Sustainable Development Goals Series

The **Sustainable Development Goals Series** is Springer Nature's inaugural cross-imprint book series that addresses and supports the United Nations' seventeen Sustainable Development Goals. The series fosters comprehensive research focused on these global targets and endeavours to address some of society's greatest grand challenges. The SDGs are inherently multidisciplinary, and they bring people working across different fields together and working towards a common goal. In this spirit, the Sustainable Development Goals series is the first at Springer Nature to publish books under both the Springer and Palgrave Macmillan imprints, bringing the strengths of our imprints together.

The Sustainable Development Goals Series is organized into eighteen subseries: one subseries based around each of the seventeen respective Sustainable Development Goals, and an eighteenth subseries, "Connecting the Goals", which serves as a home for volumes addressing multiple goals or studying the SDGs as a whole. Each subseries is guided by an expert Subseries Advisor with years or decades of experience studying and addressing core components of their respective Goal.

The SDG Series has a remit as broad as the SDGs themselves, and contributions are welcome from scientists, academics, policymakers, and researchers working in fields related to any of the seventeen goals. If you are interested in contributing a monograph or curated volume to the series, please contact the Publishers: Zachary Romano [Springer; zachary.romano@springer.com] and Rachael Ballard [Palgrave Macmillan; rachael.ballard@palgrave.com].

Valeska Padovese • Isotta Rossoni
Editors

Intersections of Sexual Health, Migration and Sexualised Violence

A Public Health and Rights-based Approach

Springer

Editors
Valeska Padovese
Genitourinary Clinic, Department of Dermatology and Venereology
Mater Dei Hospital
Msida, Malta

Isotta Rossoni
Van Vollenhoven Institute -Leiden Law School
Leiden University
Leiden, The Netherlands

ISSN 2523-3084 ISSN 2523-3092 (electronic)
Sustainable Development Goals Series
ISBN 978-3-032-20706-7 ISBN 978-3-032-20707-4 (eBook)
https://doi.org/10.1007/978-3-032-20707-4

This Springer imprint is published by the registered company Springer Nature Switzerland AG
The registered company address is: Gewerbestrasse 11, 6330 Cham, Switzerland

Preface

This publication emerges from the collaborative efforts of the two editors, who met through their respective work in sexual health and sexual violence prevention. Brought together by a shared commitment to addressing complex issues at the intersection of health, rights, and migration, they found common ground in activism and fieldwork, ultimately co-founding an NGO, Bridges2Health&Rights, to further their joint action. Valeska Padovese's background in sexual health and Isotta Rossoni's focus on sexual violence prevention opened up critical conversations around the fragmented nature of current approaches, particularly in contexts shaped by migration. Despite the overlapping realities of these fields, interdisciplinary collaborations remain limited, due to rigid institutional boundaries or siloed academic disciplines.

This work aims to challenge that norm by bridging medical and social perspectives, promoting a more holistic understanding of sexual and reproductive health and rights, centered on care and justice. Migration, as a complex, global, and cross-cutting phenomenon, highlights the urgency of this integration, revealing how health outcomes are shaped not only by biology or policy but also by displacement, trauma, and resilience. Through this publication, the editors hope to foster a dialogue that transcends sectors and geographies, inviting more inclusive and intersectional approaches to sexual health and violence prevention, in migration contexts and beyond.

We are deeply grateful to all the activists, practitioners, and professionals—many of whom have directly inspired this publication, and some of whom have penned the chapters in this book—who continue to carry out invaluable work on these critical issues. Most importantly, we thank all those with lived experiences of migration, displacement, and violence, whom we have met in our personal and professional lives and continue to meet through our work. Thank you for trusting us with your stories and your knowledge. You alert us to how deeply policies and systems impact your lives, often in ways that remain invisible to those who design them. This publication is an effort to do justice to your experiences, and in a small way, contribute to meaningful policy change.

Msida, Malta — Valeska Padovese
Leiden, The Netherlands — Isotta Rossoni

Contents

Interwoven Realities: Sexualised Violence, Health, and Migration in a Changing World

1

Isotta Rossoni and Valeska Padovese

Contents

Abstract

As of April 2025, approximately 122 million people were forcibly displaced worldwide (UNHCR 2025a). War, violence, and persecution continue to act as primary push factors of displacement. With the number of interstate conflicts nearly doubling since 2010, the global landscape has seen a rise in instability, with millions fleeing their homes in search of safety (UNHCR 2025b). While at the time of writing, Israel's ongoing actions in Gaza—widely condemned for their exceptionally high civilian death toll and the use of genocidal tactics (United Nations Human Rights Council 2022)—have attracted significant media and public attention in Europe, and, globally, it is important to recognise that other regions are also experiencing severe and sustained violence. Sudan, for instance, has been embroiled in civil war since April 2023, resulting in millions of internally displaced people and refugees. The population faces a severe humanitarian crisis, including food insecurity, localised famine, and major disruptions to aid access (United Nations Office for the Coordination of Humanitarian Affairs (OCHA) 2024). According to the ACLED Conflict Index, a global assessment of conflicts based on deadliness, danger to civilians, geographic diffusion, and the number of armed groups, Palestine, Myanmar, Syria, and Mexico are among the countries most acutely impacted by violence (Raleigh and Kishi 2025).

As of April 2025, approximately 122 million people were forcibly displaced worldwide (UNHCR 2025a). War, violence, and persecution continue to act as primary push factors of displacement. With the number of interstate conflicts nearly doubling since 2010, the global landscape has seen a rise in instability, with millions fleeing their homes in search of safety

I. Rossoni (✉)
Van Vollenhoven Institute -Leiden Law School, Leiden University, Leiden, The Netherlands

V. Padovese
Genitourinary Clinic, Department of Dermatology and Venereology, Mater Dei Hospital, Msida, Malta
e-mail: valeska.padovese@gov.mt

V. Padovese, I. Rossoni (eds.), *Intersections of Sexual Health, Migration and Sexualised Violence*, Sustainable Development Goals Series, https://doi.org/10.1007/978-3-032-20707-4_1

(UNHCR 2025b). While at the time of writing, Israel's ongoing actions in Gaza—widely condemned for their exceptionally high civilian death toll and the use of genocidal tactics (United Nations Human Rights Council 2022)—have attracted significant media and public attention in Europe, and, globally, it is important to recognise that other regions are also experiencing severe and sustained violence. Sudan, for instance, has been embroiled in civil war since April 2023, resulting in millions of internally displaced people and refugees. The population faces a severe humanitarian crisis, including food insecurity, localised famine, and major disruptions to aid access (United Nations Office for the Coordination of Humanitarian Affairs (OCHA) 2024). According to the ACLED Conflict Index, a global assessment of conflicts based on deadliness, danger to civilians, geographic diffusion, and the number of armed groups, Palestine, Myanmar, Syria, and Mexico are among the countries most acutely impacted by violence (Raleigh and Kishi 2025).

The interconnection between wars, genocides, and conflicts on one hand and displacement, forced migration, sexualised violence, and sexual and reproductive health and rights (SRHR) issues on the other has long been recognised by scholarship (Freedman et al. 2022; Egli-Gany et al. 2021; Soeiro et al. 2023; Heidari and Moreno 2016). Armed conflicts fuel migration and displacement, create the conditions for violence—particularly sexualised and gender-related—to escalate, and contribute to the breakdown of essential healthcare, including sexual and reproductive services (Hedström and Herder 2023). Recent events in Gaza exemplify how health systems and their stewards can become direct targets in war, with devastating repercussions for public health and human rights. Systematic attacks on hospitals, ambulances, and medical workers have had catastrophic consequences for both patients and those providing care (Vitale et al. 2025). Healthcare workers have faced grave risks, including death, injury, and the destruction of facilities essential for life-saving interventions. This unprecedented assault on medical work not only undermines the core principles of humanitarian law but also leaves the civilian population without access to critical health services amidst ongoing conflict.

Understanding the dynamics of overlapping health, social and rights-related concerns faced by displaced populations, and the challenges confronted by professionals offering essential services is crucial for designing effective interventions that address both immediate humanitarian needs and the broader systemic causes of hardship. Against the backdrop of rapidly evolving patterns of displacement, this book aims to unpack the complex intersections of migration, sexualised violence, and health. What sets this collection apart from other publications is its interdisciplinary and cross-regional nature. The volume brings together contributions from diverse parts of the world including Europe, Africa, and the Middle East, offering a rich tapestry of perspectives in varied contexts of displacement and migration. Crucially, contributors span a wide range of professional and disciplinary backgrounds—from medical practitioners to scholars in law, criminology, and social sciences—as well as activists and practitioners working directly with affected communities. While readers will encounter the terms *migration* and *displacement* throughout the various chapters, these words encompass a host of circumstances and experiences shaped by diverse geographical contexts, as well as by their overlap with other social conditions—a complexity that contributes to the richness and depth of the book's analysis.

The work is informed by a holistic approach to health, essential in addressing the varied needs of migrant populations, particularly those affected by displacement, trauma, and sexualised violence. Unlike traditional biomedical models, which often isolate physical symptoms, holistic care recognises the overlap of physical, psychological, and social health determinants (Engel 1977; Keygnaert et al. 2015). Migrants and refugees—especially women and girls and members of the LGBTIQA+ community—are disproportionately exposed to gender-based violence (GBV) and sexualised violence (SV) both during transit and in host countries, which can result in long-term mental health conditions such as post-traumatic stress disorder (PTSD), depression, and anxiety (Freedman et al. 2022; Freedman 2016). These effects are further compounded by systemic barriers to care, including language, legal status, stigma, and culturally inappropriate services (Hacker et al. 2015).

In order to provide a holistic exploration of health and well-being in the context of migration and displacement, this volume is organised into three core sections, each examining a key dimension of the complex relationship between displacement, sexualised violence, and health. The first section focuses on access to sexual and reproductive health (SRH) services, particularly in contexts marked by legal precarity, conflict, and systemic exclusion. In Chap. 2, Fahme, Fakih, and Mumtaz describe challenges in the prevention and treatment of sexually transmitted infections (STIs), including HIV, in the Middle East and North Africa (MENA), with a focus on forcibly displaced populations. The authors present an overview of the epidemiology of HIV and other STIs, describing the availability of sexual health services (SHS) and discussing barriers to SHS accessibility. The chapter stresses that the region has the world's highest increase in HIV incidence, primarily affecting key populations, as well as a high burden of curable STIs, most likely due to limited access to screening and treatment. Although data on HIV and STIs among forcibly displaced populations in MENA remain scarce, available evidence suggests a high prevalence, mainly among refugees who are part of key populations, including men who have sex with men (MSM). Though some MENA states have integrated sexual health services into primary care settings, services remain insufficient to meet current needs. Various barriers to access persist, including conservative societal norms, fragmented health systems, prolonged conflict, and pervasive stigma around sexuality and sexual health. For refugees in MENA, who are already vulnerable to adverse sexual and reproductive health outcomes, accessing SHS poses additional challenges.

In Chap. 3, Blondeel et al. delve deeper into HPV (human papillomavirus) and access to cervical cancer screening in migrants and refugees, presenting the literature and available data on coverage, barriers, and opportunities for cervical cancer prevention among these populations. Crucially, they outline barriers to HPV vaccination and primary and secondary cervical cancer prevention, relying on an ecological model based on personal, interpersonal, organisational, structural, and contextual obstacles. Recognising that migrants face many barriers to vaccination against HPV due to the absence or disruption of vaccination systems in their countries, they highlight how updated WHO guidelines and innovations hold promise for reaching underserved women and individuals with a cervix.

Chapter 4, authored by Rossoni and Camilleri, explores the challenges faced by sex workers, particularly those with a migrant background, in accessing healthcare and ancillary services in Malta, a small Southern European country at the crossroads between Africa and Europe. The authors draw on qualitative data, centred around the lived experiences of sex workers. Inspired by Levesque et al.'s "access to healthcare" framework (Levesque et al. 2013), they explore the different dimensions of access to health—including following experiences of violence from the perspectives of individuals selling sexual services. The findings highlight that migrant sex workers generally face substantial barriers in accessing sexual health services, especially after experiencing violence. These include strict residency and taxation requirements for HIV treatment, reliance on private healthcare due to delays in public health services, and biases among healthcare practitioners related to sex work, gender, and race. These biases can significantly impact access to dignified care, particularly in cases of sexual and other violence experienced during sex work. The chapter emphasises the need for policy reforms to improve healthcare access for sex workers and targeted training for professionals on working with migrant sex workers. The authors further advocate for research into the role of peer education in improving access to health services.

In Chap. 5, Enbiale describes sexual and reproductive health challenges in the African context. Africa faces one of the world's largest internal displacement crises, with over 35 million people internally displaced due to conflict and related disruptions in social, economic, and healthcare systems. Women and girls are disproportionately affected, facing unique sexual health challenges, alongside high percentages of preventable maternal, neonatal, and under-five deaths. Sexual violence is prevalent, exacerbated by limited humanitarian access and inadequate survivor support, including post-exposure prophylaxis (PEP) and emergency contraception. Key barriers include limited contraception access (IDP women have double the unmet family planning needs), lack of skilled birth attendants, and insufficiently integrated GBV healthcare services. Displacement disrupts supply chains, restricting condoms, pre-exposure prophylaxis (PrEP), and post-exposure prophylaxis (PEP) availability. Healthcare worker shortages and stigma around STIs further impede diagnosis and treatment. Community education programmes are often deprioritised during crises, leaving displaced populations uninformed about prevention and symptom recognition. The author recommends integrating sexual health into primary care with trained frontline workers, mobile clinics, telehealth, and strengthened referral systems to improve survivor outcomes. Culturally sensitive outreach programmes could also help encourage awareness and access to sexual health services. Yet, long-term solutions require policy reforms, increased government funding, and survivor-centred care models to combat stigma and systemic barriers.

Building on the exploration of the multifaceted barriers to healthcare access faced by different groups within the migrant population in diverse geographical settings, the second section of the book shifts the focus to the health outcomes experienced by displaced populations, examining physical, mental, and emotional impacts. Chapter 6, by O'Doherty, synthesises research on the experiences and outcomes of migrant survivors of sexual violence, highlighting their unique challenges in accessing care and the need for trauma-informed, culturally sensitive responses. Sexual violence is a pervasive issue intricately linked to migration, with profound health and well-being consequences for survivors. Sexual and gender-based violence acts as both a cause and risk factor throughout migration journeys. Many migrate to escape violence, including sexualised violence, which escalates during conflict and displacement. Migrants, particularly children and young people in overcrowded refugee camps, face heightened risks of abuse and exploitation during transit and post-migration. On top of this, policy measures aimed at controlling migration may also, inadvertently, generate vulnerabilities. Moreover, the persistence of gender-based abuse shifts perpetrators and abuse types during migration phases—from opportunistic violence during transit to domestic abuse post-migration. The author advocates for better access to safe housing, health services, legal protections, and social support: all these aspects critically influence survivors' risks and recovery.

In Chap. 7, Admassu et al. explore the complex relationships between intimate partner violence (IPV), sexual relationship power, and depression among urban refugee youth in Kampala, Uganda. Their work emphasises the disproportionate impact of intimate partner violence (IPV) and depression on refugee youth and investigates how sexual relationship power mediates the effect of IPV on depression, aiming to inform targeted interventions for mental health and relationship dynamics in this vulnerable population. IPV, encompassing physical, sexual, or psychological harm by a partner, affects about one-third of women globally and is strongly linked to adverse health outcomes, including mental health disorders such as depression, anxiety, and PTSD. Refugee youth face heightened risks due to factors like food insecurity, poverty, disrupted family roles, and trauma, which exacerbate IPV risk and mental health challenges. Drawing on research conducted with over 300 refugee youth aged 16–24 years, reporting experiences of IPV, the authors find that depression severity varies among participants. The chapter confirms that urban refugee youth experiencing IPV report diminished sexual relationship power and increased depression, in line with prior research in similar contexts. The research underscores the need for gender-transformative, youth-centred interventions that address sexual relationship power and IPV prevention to promote mental health among refugee youth. Collaborative approaches involving local stakeholders and refugee youth themselves are crucial for culturally relevant programming.

In Chap. 8, Bartovic et al. provide a lucid analysis of the health consequences of immigration detention. The confinement of individuals for migration-related procedures, otherwise known as immigration detention, is increasingly used worldwide despite international legal standards that provide it should be the last resort. This practice encompasses a wide range of facility types and conditions, often varying by country, with significant differences in detention duration, legal oversight, and the treatment of vulnerable populations such as children and families. Detention conditions vary widely, impacting the health and well-being of detainees, including children and LGBTQIA+ individuals. Poor living conditions, overcrowding and inadequate health services contribute to a decline in health over time. Communicable diseases, such as respiratory and dermatological infections, are prevalent due to overcrowding and poor hygiene, with the COVID-19 pandemic exacerbating these risks. Non-communicable diseases may also worsen in detention, and physical injuries and abuse are significant concerns. The authors emphasise that women and children face particular health risks, which include high rates of mental health disorders, inadequate maternity care, nutritional deficits, and reproductive rights violations for women; and developmental delays, exacerbation of health conditions, missed immunisations, and severe mental health impacts often persisting post-release for children. Mental health issues are also widespread among detainees, with high prevalence of depression, anxiety, PTSD, sleep disorders, and instances of self-harm and suicide attempts. Stressors include uncertainty about detention duration, legal confusion, lack of autonomy, mistreatment by staff, isolation, and substandard conditions.

The authors conclude that the detention environment is a critical determinant of poor health outcomes and increased risks of sexual and gender-based violence among refugees and migrants. Despite international legal prohibitions and the documented harms, immigration detention remains widely used, with many facilities failing to meet the required standards. This overview highlights the urgent need to prioritise alternatives to detention and implement comprehensive harm reduction strategies.

The final section of the book brings the discussion full circle by focusing on prevention and response from the perspective of health professionals working with migrants and refugees, while also exploring the possibilities offered by novel technologies. Despite the demanding nature of high-stress environments like humanitarian settings, the experiences of healthcare workers remain underexplored. Those working in humanitarian settings face a multitude of risks that threaten their safety, well-being, and ability to provide care. They are frequently exposed to violence in the form of physical assault, kidnapping, or intimidation by combatants or criminal groups (Nickerson 2015). The constant threat of violence, coupled with witnessing severe injuries or deaths, and the pressure to deliver care under resource-constrained conditions, contribute to high levels of stress, burnout, and mental health challenges such as anxiety, depression, and post-traumatic stress disorder (Cameron et al. 2024). The physical health of healthcare workers is also at risk due to poor living and working conditions, long hours, and limited access to nutritious food and clean water.

Resource scarcity is another significant challenge, as there is often a lack of essential medical supplies, medicines, and equipment, forcing healthcare workers to make difficult decisions about rationing care, which can lead to moral distress and ethical dilemmas (Broussard et al. 2019). In addition to this, navigating complex local laws, cultural norms and humanitarian principles may expose them to legal jeopardy or professional censure and even to social exclusion from local communities, especially if perceived as outsiders or as contravening prevailing social or political norms (Rubenstein and Haar 2022). For female healthcare workers and those from marginalised groups, there is also a heightened risk of sexual and gender-based violence, including harassment, assault, or exploitation in insecure environments (Murphy et al. 2024).

In Chap. 9, Jachmann expands upon these issues, identifying the challenges and necessary support mechanisms for volunteer and professional aid workers providing care to migrants and refugees, especially survivors of sexual violence. Jachmann highlights the high levels of stress and the complex demands faced by aid workers, emphasising the importance of tailored training and mental health support to enhance their competence, resilience, and well-being. She teases out the impacts of stress at the personal level—in terms of private life, relationships, mental, and physical health—and at the organisational/systemic level. Jachmann stresses the need for specialised training for healthcare professionals, intersectoral collaboration, networking, good teamwork, and communication to ensure workers' well-being and, in turn, better address the complex needs of migrants and refugees. The chapter offers useful tips and guidelines to ensure that appropriate professional pathways are designed for healthcare professionals working with these populations.

Shifting the focus from human capital to technology in service of marginalised communities, in Chap. 10, Padovese et al. examine how POCT and NPT can play a transformative role in STI prevention and treatment among populations that are often underserved by mainstream health services. Effective sexual and reproductive healthcare for displaced and marginalised populations hinges on innovative strategies to bridge access gaps and address unique barriers faced by these groups. Timely and accurate diagnosis of sexually transmitted infections (STIs) is crucial, not only for individual health but also for broader public health, given the rise of antimicrobial resistance and the challenges posed by traditional clinic-based testing. The chapter discusses how these technologies can facilitate rapid diagnosis and prompt treatment, which is particularly important in the context of increasing antimicrobial resistance. By enabling immediate results and reducing delays between testing and treatment, POCT helps to ensure that infections are managed appropriately, minimising the misuse of antibiotics and curbing the spread of resistant strains. Moreover, accessible and community-based STI testing empowers individuals to seek care without fear of stigma or discrimination, ultimately supporting both individual well-being and public health goals.

Community-based and culturally sensitive testing reduces the fear and shame often associated with clinic-based STI services especially if delivered with the support of peer educators or cultural mediators helping bridge the cultural and linguistic gap. The authors also highlight the cost effectiveness of outreach interventions combined to community testing. POCT is economically viable, especially when integrated into broader community health programmes. STI testing should be bundled with other health services (e.g. HIV, hepatitis, TB) to maximise reach and efficiency. Mobile clinics, vending machines, and outreach programmes bring testing closer to "hard-to-reach populations", support early detection, and reduce transmission aligning with global health goals for STI elimination. Moreover, they ensure quality assurance, avoid over-reliance on unvalidated tests, and maintain ethical standards in data handling and patient confidentiality.

Across the volume, authors writing from diverse experiences, disciplines, and regional contexts collectively underscore the multifaceted sexual and reproductive health challenges faced by displaced populations. Migration flows are complex in that they encompass a variety of experiences and individuals, including asylum-seekers, refugees, stateless persons, trafficked persons, unaccompanied/separated children, smuggled migrants, and migrants in an irregular situation. Each group has different protection needs and entitlements, though some overlap and categories are rarely fixed. When refugees and asylum-seekers move in mixed flows, their international protection needs may not be identified, and they may be at higher risk of refoulement. Irregularised migrants are frequently excluded from mainstream health services and vulnerable to exploitation and unsafe working conditions. They can endure considerable mental and physical health challenges, exacerbated by social isolation, fear of detention, and barriers to preventive and emergency care. These complexities further underscore the importance of adopting comprehensive, inclusive approaches to migrant health that address the unique needs of all individuals on the move. Whilst acknowledging these overarching needs, it is also crucial to recognise the specific vulnerabilities faced by marginalised subgroups such as women and girls, sex workers, and LGBTIQA+ individuals.

Though the issues at hand are undeniably complex and require multilayered responses involving education, empowerment, training, and sustainable resource allocation, a common thread throughout the book is the call for humane, person-centred, and intersectional policy solutions. These must move beyond reactive frameworks to embrace a holistic view of health that recognises the interdependence of physical, sexual, emotional, and psychological well-being. Crucially, the book advocates for policies that are informed by the lived experiences of displaced individuals and those who work alongside them, ensuring that reforms are not only effective but also grounded in the realities of those most affected.

References

Broussard G, Rubenstein LS, Robinson C, Gagnon AJ, Delaunay S, Borcard E et al (2019) Challenges to ethical obligations and humanitarian principles in conflict settings: a systematic review. Int J Humanit Action 4:15. https://doi.org/10.1186/s41018-019-0063-x

Cameron L, McCauley M, van den Broek N, McCauley H (2024) The occurrence of and factors associated with mental ill-health amongst humanitarian aid workers: a systematic review and meta-analysis. PLoS One 19(5):e0292107. https://doi.org/10.1371/journal.pone.0292107

Egli-Gany D, Aftab W, Hawkes S, Abu-Raddad L, Buse K, Rabbani F, Low N, Onarheim K (2021) The social and structural determinants of sexual and reproductive health and rights in migrants and refugees: a systematic review of reviews. East Mediterr Health J 27(12):1232–1242

Engel GL (1977) The need for a new medical model: a challenge for biomedicine. Science 196(4286):129–136

Freedman J (2016) Sexual and gender-based violence against refugee women: a hidden aspect of the refugee "crisis". Reprod Health Matters 24(47):18–26

Freedman J, Sahraoui N, Tastsoglou E (2022) Gender-based violence in migration: interdisciplinary, feminist and intersectional approaches. Springer, Cham

Hacker K, Anies M, Folb BL, Zallman L (2015) Barriers to health care for undocumented immigrants: a literature review. Risk Manag Healthc Policy 8:175–183

Hedström J, Herder T (2023) Women's sexual and reproductive health in war and conflict: are we seeing the full picture? Glob Health Action 16(1):2188689. https://doi.org/10.1080/16549716.2023.2188689

Heidari S, Moreno CG (2016) Gender-based violence: a barrier to sexual and reproductive health and rights. Reprod Health Matters 24(47):1–4. https://doi.org/10.1016/j.rhm.2016.07.001

Keygnaert I, Ivanova O, Guieu A, Van Parys AS, Leye E, Roelens K (2015) What is the evidence on the reduction of gender-based violence in humanitarian and development contexts? Health evidence network synthesis report 57 [Internet]. WHO Regional Office for Europe, Copenhagen. [cited 2025 Oct 6]. Available from: https://www.euro.who.int/__data/assets/pdf_file/0011/291636/HEN-synthesis-report-57.pdf

Levesque JF, Harris MF, Russell G (2013) Patient-centred access to health care: conceptualising access at the interface of health systems and populations. Int J Equity Health 12:18. https://doi.org/10.1186/1475-9276-12-18

Murphy M, Potts A, Nassif G, Khalfallah LA, Kaisi J, Modi AT et al (2024) Violence against women and girls in conflict: progress and priorities. Lancet 404(10471):2495–2498. https://doi.org/10.1016/S0140-6736(23)02783-1

Nickerson JW (2015) Ensuring the security of health care in conflict settings: an urgent global health concern. CMAJ 187(11):E347–E348. https://doi.org/10.1503/cmaj.140410. PMID: 25991837; PMCID: PMC4527929

Raleigh C, Kishi K (2025) Conflict index [Internet]. ACLED; [cited 2025 Oct 6]. Available from: https://acleddata.com/series/acled-conflict-index

Rubenstein L, Haar R (2022) What does ethics demand of health care practice in conflict zones? AMA J Ethics 24(6):E535–E541. https://doi.org/10.1001/amajethics.2022.535

Soeiro RE, de Siqueira Guida JP, da-Costa-Santos J, Costa ML (2023) Sexual and reproductive health (SRH) needs for forcibly displaced adolescent girls and young women (10–24 years old) in humanitarian settings: a mixed-methods systematic review. Reprod Health 20(1):174. https://doi.org/10.1186/s12978-023-01715-8. PMID: 37996929; PMCID: PMC10668438

UNHCR (2025a) Displacement overview – April 2025 snapshot [Internal mid-year update]. United Nations High Commissioner for Refugees, Geneva

UNHCR (2025b) More than 123 million people forcibly displaced by end of 2024, UNHCR says [Internet]. Euronews. [cited 2025 Oct 5]. Available from: https://www.euronews.com/2025/06/12/more-than-123-million-people-forcibly-displaced-by-end-of-2024-unhcr-says

United Nations Human Rights Council (2022) Report of the human rights council on its sixtieth session. United Nations, Geneva. Available from: https://www.ohchr.org/sites/default/files/documents/hrbodies/hrcouncil/sessions-regular/session60/advance-version/a-hrc-60-crp-3.pdf

United Nations Office for the Coordination of Humanitarian Affairs (OCHA). Sudan: A two-year crisis through the lens of a photo-journalist [Internet]. 2024. [cited 2025 Oct 15]. Available from: http://unocha.org/news/sudan-two-year-crisis-through-lens-photojournalist

Vitale A, Pizzol D, Ceschi A (2025) Gaza's healthocide: medical societies must not stay silent. Lancet 406(10511):1467–1468

HIV and Sexually Transmitted Infections in the Middle East and North Africa: Stigma and Other Access Barriers to Sexual Health Services Among Forcibly Displaced Populations

2

Sasha A. Fahme, Iman Fakih, and Ghina R. Mumtaz

Contents

Abstract

This chapter describes the main challenges in the prevention and treatment of sexually transmitted infections (STIs), including HIV, in the Middle East and North Africa (MENA), with a focus on forcibly displaced populations. It presents an overview of the epidemiology of HIV and other STIs, describes the availability of sexual health services (SHS), and discusses barriers to SHS accessibility. MENA has the world's highest increase in HIV incidence, primarily affecting key populations. The region also has a high burden of curable STIs, most

S. A. Fahme
Center for Global Health, Weill Cornell Medicine, New York, NY, USA

I. Fakih
Department of Epidemiology and Population Health, American University of Beirut, Beirut, Lebanon

G. R. Mumtaz (✉)
Department of Epidemiology and Population Health, American University of Beirut, Beirut, Lebanon

Center for Infectious Diseases Research, Faculty of Medicine, American University of Beirut, Beirut, Lebanon
e-mail: gm15@aub.edu.lb

V. Padovese, I. Rossoni (eds.), *Intersections of Sexual Health, Migration and Sexualised Violence*, Sustainable Development Goals Series, https://doi.org/10.1007/978-3-032-20707-4_2

likely due to limited access to screening and treatment. Data on HIV and STIs among forcibly displaced populations in MENA are scarce, but suggest high prevalence mainly among refugees who are part of key populations, including men who have sex with men. Though some MENA states have integrated SHS into primary care settings, services remain insufficient to meet current needs. Various barriers to access persist, including conservative societal norms, fragmented health systems, prolonged conflict, and pervasive stigma around sexuality and sexual health. For refugees in MENA, who are already vulnerable to adverse sexual and reproductive health outcomes, accessing SHS poses additional challenges. A multifaceted approach is urgently needed to meet the region's evolving STI disease burden and sexual health needs, including among its large forcibly displaced population.

Keywords

HIV · Sexually transmitted infections · Sexual health services · Stigma · Forcibly displaced populations · Refugees · Middle East and North Africa

Abbreviations

ART	Antiretroviral therapy
FSW	Female sex worker
HBV	Hepatitis B virus
HPV	Human papilloma virus
MENA	Middle East and North Africa
MSM	Men who have sex with men
NGO	Non-governmental organization
PHC	Primary healthcare centre
PLHIV	People living with HIV
PWID	People who inject drugs
SHS	Sexual health services
STI	Sexually transmitted infection
UAE	United Arab Emirates
UNAIDS	Joint United Nations Programme on HIV/AIDS
UNHCR	United Nations High Commissioner for Refugees
UNRWA	United Nations Relief and Works Agency for Palestine Refugees in the Near East
VCT	Voluntary counselling and testing
WHO	World Health Organization

2.1 Introduction

Sexually transmitted infections (STIs), including HIV, have been historically neglected by policy makers in the Middle East and North Africa (MENA). The complexities of addressing STIs are compounded in this region by conservative societal norms and sensitivities surrounding sexuality (Abu-Raddad et al. 2010a, b, 2013). While it has often been believed that there are no reliable data on STIs in MENA, there have been significant improvements in our understanding of regional STI epidemiology in the last decade (Abu-Raddad et al. 2010b, c, 2013; Chemaitelly et al. 2019a, b; Harfouche et al. 2023; Mumtaz et al. 2010, 2014a, b, 2022; Saba et al. 2013; Smolak et al. 2019; World Health Organization 2024a). However, the public health response remains insufficient to address the current disease burden and the sexual health needs of affected populations (World Health Organization 2024a).

Despite global advancements in STI prevention and treatment strategies, the MENA region continues to face barriers to effectively curbing the spread of STIs and providing comprehensive sexual health services (SHS) (World Health Organization 2024a). Progress has been hampered by challenges such as heterogeneous data availability and quality across the region, restrictive social norms, pervasive stigma, and insufficient SHS infrastructure, among others. These obstacles not only affect prevention efforts but also impact the provision of care and support for people living with HIV (PLHIV) and other STIs.

Over the past 15 years, the MENA region has also experienced substantial sociopolitical and economic crises resulting in massive forced displacement. These humanitarian crises have implications for the transmission and control of STIs including HIV, further exacerbating the already-fragile response to this disease burden (Mumtaz et al. 2022). By the end of 2022, approximately half of the global refugee population originated from countries that are part of the MENA region (UNHCR 2023).

Refugees from Syria remain the largest forcibly displaced population globally, accounting for 20% of all refugees and other people in need of protection (UNHCR 2023). They have been living in protracted displacement since 2011. Refugees from Afghanistan, another MENA country, rank third among global refugee populations, with an estimated 5.3 million refugees and asylum seekers fleeing poverty, hunger, recurrent natural disasters, and widespread human rights violations following decades of conflict (UNHCR 2023). The majority of the global refugee population is resettled in neighbouring low- and middle-income countries (UNHCR 2023). Afghan refugees are mainly hosted in bordering Iran and Pakistan (UNHCR 2023). Lebanon and Jordan, two MENA countries, host the largest per-capita number of refugees in the world—primarily from Syria and Palestine—with one in four individuals in each of these two countries being a refugee (UNHCR 2023).

Several factors contribute to poor sexual health outcomes in humanitarian settings. The delivery of health services is frequently disrupted, and humanitarian agencies face challenges in meeting even the most basic needs of affected populations (Starrs et al. 2018). Under such strained conditions, sexual and reproductive health needs are often overlooked and inadequately prioritized (Panchenko et al. 2024). Additionally, there is a documented increase in structural determinants of HIV and STI transmission, including poverty, food insecurity, and trauma, all of which disproportionately impact women, rendering them more susceptible to sexual and gender-based violence and to engaging in transactional sex to secure essential resources for their families (Hankins et al. 2002). A growing body of literature and humanitarian reports suggest the presence of transactional sex work, early marriage, and sex trafficking among refugee women in MENA (Trafficking in Persons Report 2017; Yasmine and Moughalian 2016; Charles and Denman 2013; Samari 2017; Bartels et al. 2018; Bartels and Hamill 2014).

This chapter aims at providing a general understanding of the challenges and opportunities in addressing STIs including HIV in the MENA region, with a specific focus on forcibly displaced populations. We present an overview of the epidemiology of HIV and other STIs, describe the availability of and access to SHS, and discuss barriers to SHS accessibility highlighting the role of stigma within the context of humanitarian settings.

Our definition of MENA includes 24 countries that are part of the MENA definitions of the three international organizations leading most HIV/AIDS and STIs efforts in this region—the Joint United Nations Programme on HIV/AIDS (UNAIDS), the World Health Organization (WHO), and the World Bank (Fig. 2.1). The

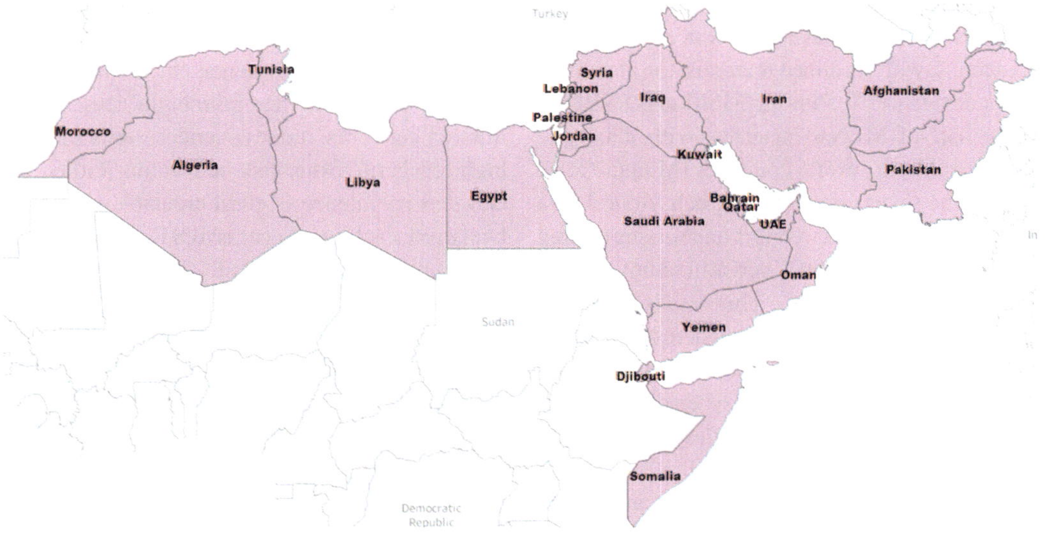

Fig. 2.1 Map of the Middle East and North Africa region

countries are Afghanistan, Algeria, Bahrain, Djibouti, Egypt, Iran, Iraq, Jordan, Kuwait, Lebanon, Libya, Morocco, Oman, Pakistan, Palestine, Qatar, Saudi Arabia, Somalia, Sudan, South Sudan, Syria, Tunisia, United Arab Emirates, and Yemen. Together, these countries account for 11% of the world's population (Population Reference Bureau 2024).

2.2 HIV and STIs Epidemiology in MENA

2.2.1 HIV Epidemiology

The prevalence of HIV among the general population is well below 1% in all MENA countries except for Djibouti, Somalia, and South Sudan where the HIV epidemics share epidemiological characteristics with neighbouring sub-Saharan Africa (Abu-Raddad et al. 2010b). Still, MENA is one of only three world regions where HIV incidence is on the rise and is the region with the highest increase in incidence (61% since 2010) (UNAIDS 2023a). In MENA, most HIV transmission occurs among key populations, including people who inject drugs (PWID), men who have sex with men (MSM), female sex workers (FSWs), and their sexual partners (UNAIDS 2023a).

Indeed, there is a documented trend of increasing HIV prevalence among the three key populations in MENA (Mumtaz et al. 2022). The evidence indicates persistent concentrated HIV epidemics, with sustained transmission at considerable levels (>5%), among MSM and PWID in about half of MENA countries with data, and among FSWs in several countries (Mumtaz et al. 2022). The sexual and injecting behavioural data indicate a high-risk environment, suggesting potential for further HIV spread (Mumtaz et al. 2010, 2014a, 2018, 2022). There is also substantial overlap of risk behaviours across the three key populations, which appears to have contributed to the observed patterns of epidemic emergence over the past two decades (Chemaitelly et al. 2019b; Mumtaz et al. 2010, 2014a, 2018, 2022). However, data gaps persist in several countries, precluding a characterization of the status of the HIV epidemic and suggesting the possibility of hidden epidemics in these settings (Mumtaz et al. 2022).

2.2.2 STI Epidemiology

A recent comprehensive assessment of STI epidemiology in the Eastern Mediterranean region (all MENA countries defined above except for Algeria and South Sudan) documented a substantial and largely overlooked STI disease burden (World Health Organization 2024a; Smolak et al. 2019). The prevalence of curable STIs in the general population was determined to be comparable to global levels at 3.1% for chlamydia, 1.9% for gonorrhoea, 0.4% for syphilis, and 4.6% for trichomoniasis (World Health Organization 2024a; Smolak et al. 2019). A higher prevalence of chlamydia and gonorrhoea was found among infertility clinic attendees and women with ectopic pregnancies and miscarriages, reflecting the morbidity of untreated STIs and their contribution to adverse reproductive outcomes in this region (World Health Organization 2024a; Smolak et al. 2019). This is in contrast with the low prevalence of chlamydia and gonorrhoea observed among these population groups in countries of the global North, such as in Europe, with robust and well-established sexual health and STI programs (Eggert-Kruse et al. 1996, 2011; Dietrich et al. 2010; Miron et al. 2013; Chemaitelly et al. 2021).

While the high prevalence of curable STIs in the region suggests the presence of active transmission networks, it does not necessarily indicate high levels of sexual risk behaviour. Rather, the elevated prevalence of these treatable infections likely reflects limited access to STI screening and treatment services. Indeed, the prevalence of chronic viral STIs such as herpes simplex virus type 2, estimated at 5.1% in the general population (World Health Organization 2024a), is overall lower in MENA than in other world regions (Abu-Raddad et al. 2010a, b; Harfouche et al. 2023; Mumtaz et al. 2022; Vaccarella et al. 2013; Dargham et al. 2018).

2.2.3 HIV and STIs Epidemiology Among Forcibly Displaced Populations

Despite an increase in the social and structural determinants of HIV and STI transmission and severity in humanitarian settings, data on the impact of conflict and displacement on STI incidence and prevalence are not consistent in the global literature. In some settings in Sub-Saharan Africa, lower HIV prevalence was found in conflict-affected populations, which may be due to a decline in mobility and urbanization during periods of war (Abu-Raddad et al. 2010c). Yet, such conditions may not be applicable to MENA, where millions of displaced people have settled over the years in urban settings within neighbouring countries (Guterres and Spiegel 2012; Fawaz et al. 2021; Jauhiainen and Eyvazlu 2018).

Data on the prevalence of HIV and other STIs among forcibly displaced populations in MENA are scarce. The few available estimates suggest high prevalence among refugees who are part of key populations, while suggesting a lower burden of STIs among general population groups such as pregnant women. For example, concentrated HIV and hepatitis B virus (HBV) epidemics, with prevalence rates of 5.9% and 9.1% respectively, were observed among Afghan refugees in Pakistan, specifically within the context of high drug injection use (Khanani et al. 2010). Similarly, the prevalence of HIV among a sample of Syrian, Palestinian, and Iraqi refugee MSM in Lebanon was found to be 2.7%, with high levels of sexual-risk behaviour reported including sex work and low condom use (Tohme et al. 2016a). In contrast, no cases of HIV, syphilis, or HBV were found in a sample of Syrian and Palestinian refugee women in Lebanon (Abi Zaki et al. 2020). A very low prevalence of 0.5% for chlamydia, 0.2% for trichomoniasis, and 0.0% for gonorrhoea was also detected among pregnant Syrian refugee women in Lebanon, a low-risk population mainly engaged in monogamous sexual partnerships in the context of marriage (Fahme et al. 2024).

2.3 Sexual Health Services in MENA

2.3.1 General Overview of SHS in MENA

The MENA region has the poorest performance of all WHO regions on all key HIV response indicators, falling short of achieving the 95-95-95 global targets for HIV testing, treatment, and viral suppression (Table 2.1) (UNAIDS 2023a; World Health Organization 2023).

In 2022, only 38% of PLHIV in MENA were aware of their status, 27% had access to antiretroviral therapy (ART), and 24% were virally suppressed (World Health Organization 2023). None of the 24 countries achieved the global targets for HIV testing, and in half of countries with data, still less than 50% of PLHIV know their status (Table 2.1). The vast majority of countries are still far from achieving the global targets for treatment, and very few have data on viral suppression (Table 2.1). Just two countries—Kuwait and Saudi Arabia—have achieved the ART and viral suppression targets, though ART coverage remains insufficient in the remainder of the region.

As with HIV, other STIs remain neglected in national public health agendas in the MENA (Taylor et al. 2022). Less than half of MENA countries have a national strategy plan for STI prevention and control (UNAIDS 2023b), and only four have implemented STI surveillance systems (Taylor et al. 2022). Routine syphilis screening in pregnancy is instituted in only half of the countries (UNAIDS 2023b). While human papilloma virus (HPV) vaccination is included in the national immunization program of seven countries, primarily high-income Gulf Cooperation Council countries, just 2% of eligible girls had received one-dose coverage by the end of 2022 (World Health Organization 2024b).

The provision of essential SHS, including HIV services, within primary healthcare centres (PHCs) remains a key strategy to ensure comprehensive and universally accessibly services. An assessment of the integration of SHS into PHCs across 11 Arab countries in MENA was done in

Table 2.1 HIV treatment cascade in 2022 for countries in the MENA region (UNAIDS 2024)

	PLHIV who know their status	PLHIV on treatment	PLHIV who are virally supressed
Afghanistan	27% [10–100%]	9% [4–37%]	6% [2–25%]
Algeria	79% [73–85%]	63% [58–68%]	–
Bahrain	–	–	–
Djibouti	–	–	–
Egypt	74% [64–85%]	47% [41–55%]	39% [34–45%]
Iran	51% [39–72%]	37% [28–51%]	33% [25–46%]
Iraq	43% [32–69%]	30% [23–49%]	–
Jordan	65% [57–73%]	50% [44–56%]	47% [41–53%]
Kuwait	94 [85->98%]	93% [84->98%]	93 [83->98%]
Lebanon	86% [72->98%]	80% [67–94%]	76% [63–89%]
Libya	–	65% [58–71%]	–
Morocco	79% [72–89%]	74% [68–84%]	69% [63–78%]
Occupied Palestinian territory	–	–	–
Oman	85% [78–90%]	71% [65–75%]	64% [59–68%]
Pakistan	–	13% [12–14%]	–
Qatar	58% [42–80%]	41% [30–57%]	40% [29–55%]
Saudi Arabia	91% [83->98%]	90% [82->98%]	89% [82->98%]
Somalia	–	–	–
South Sudan		32% [26–41%]	
Sudan	48% [40–58%]	28% [23–33%]	–
Syria	78% [62–99%]	51% [41–65%]	–
Tunisia	–	26% [19–37%]	24% [17–34%]
United Arab Emirates	49% [40–59%]	47% [39–57%]	–
Yemen	52% [49–54%]	39% [37–41%]	–

MENA Middle East and North Africa, *PLHIV* people living with HIV

2017–2018 by Kabakian-Kasholian et al. (Kabakian-Khasholian et al. 2020) and portrays a grim picture (Table 2.2).

While most of the Arab countries provide STI screening, diagnosis, and treatment at the level of PHC, only Morocco, Oman, Tunisia, and the United Arab Emirates (UAE) provide the vast majority of SHS (Table 2.2). Additionally, only Morocco and Oman provide the four essential HIV services at the PHC level, followed closely by Tunisia and the UAE which provide three out of the four essential HIV services (Table 2.2). Yet, these countries fall short of meeting the global HIV targets (Table 2.1). In the case of Tunisia, only around a quarter of PLWH are on treatment and are virally suppressed (UNAIDS 2024), despite good integration of SHS into PHC (Kabakian-Khasholian et al. 2020), suggesting widespread barriers to accessing the services.

Non-governmental organizations (NGOs) play a crucial role in SHS delivery, particularly for hard-to-reach and key populations, in multiple MENA countries. Close partnerships with local NGOs enable governments to effectively channel their HIV response within socio-culturally sensitive contexts. This has been a successful model in both Lebanon and Morocco, where NGOs serve as entry point for most affected communities and are equipped to deliver comprehensive SHS (Abu-Raddad et al. 2010c).

2.3.2 SHS Among Forcibly Displaced Populations

Refugees and other forcibly displaced populations may face additional barriers to SHS accessibility. For Palestinian refugees in the region, SHS are not explicitly listed under services provided by the United Nations Relief and Works Agency for Palestine Refugees in the Near East (UNRWA), the agency tasked with providing care for Palestinian refugees (UNRWA 2024). While reproductive health services, including family planning services, are provided in UNRWA-operated PHCs, SHS, specifically STI prevention and treatment, are not listed among

Table 2.2 Essential sexual health services provided at primary health care in 11 Arab countries of MENA

	STIs/RTIs screening, diagnosis and treatment	Cervical cancer screening	Prevention and management of gender-based violence	Essential HIV services (number available out of 4[a])
Egypt				2
Jordan	✓		✓	1
Lebanon	✓	✓	✓	0
Libya				0
Morocco	✓	✓	✓	4
Oman	✓	✓		4
Palestine	✓	✓	✓	1
KSA				1
Sudan	✓			2
Tunisia	✓	✓	✓	3
UAE	✓	✓	✓	3

Adapted from Kabakian-Kasholian et al. (2020)
MENA Middle East and North Africa, *STIs* Sexually transmitted Infections, *RTIs* Reproductive Tract Infections, *UAE* United Arab Emirates
[a]The four essential HIV services selected are HIV counselling and testing, antiretroviral therapy, condom provision, and psycho-social support

the official services provided by the agency (UNRWA 2024; McCall et al. 2023).

Improving access to healthcare for Syrian refugees in the region remains a multifaceted challenge, with sexual health often overlooked. In Lebanon, various entities including the Ministry of Public Health, the United Nations High Commissioner for Refugees (UNHCR), and local and international NGOs, strive to offer subsidized healthcare services within the local healthcare system (Yassin 2018; APIS Health Consulting Group 2016). However, due to limited registration with UNHCR, approximately 75% of Syrian refugees in Lebanon must bear the full burden of medical expenses, unless they are privately insured (Lebanon 2020). It is thus unsurprising that uptake of both sexual and reproductive health services is low in this population (McCall et al. 2023). A recent qualitative study conducted with stakeholders in Lebanon revealed a significant unmet need among adolescent Syrian refugee girls, particularly concerning adolescent pregnancy, reproductive tract infections, and gender-based violence (Fahme et al. 2021).

A comparable situation exists in Jordan. Despite the provision of free primary healthcare by the Ministry of Public Health for Syrian refugees, and substantial humanitarian aid dedicated to refugee reproductive health, there are notable gaps in awareness and access (Samari 2017). A recent survey found that around one-fifth of refugee women in camps were not aware of available SRH services, and approximately one-quarter had unplanned pregnancies (Samari 2017).

Similar challenges in the provision of and access to SHS exist for Afghan refugees, the second largest refugee population in MENA and the third largest in the world (UNHCR 2023). It is estimated that Iran and Pakistan each host over three million Afghan refugees, with only 23% in Iran (UNHCR n.d.-a) and 46% in Pakistan (Gluck 2023) being registered with the UNHCR, which further complicates their access to health services. In Iran, primary health care is provided free of charge for refugees, as it is to locals (Zakian Khorramabadi et al. 2023). SRH services are integrated into Iran's primary healthcare network and include antenatal and postnatal care, family planning, as well as STI prevention. However, midwives, who are typically the primary providers of SHS to women, often lack training in sexual health counselling, leading to inadequate service provision (Rostamkhani et al. 2015; Mohseni et al. 2023). Further, Afghan refugees in Iran report instances of discrimination and substandard treatment, potentially impacting the quality of care they receive (Heydari et al. 2016).

In Pakistan, healthcare coverage for refugees varies based on their place of residence and the type of care required. Pakistan's national health system covers all healthcare (essential, secondary, and tertiary care) for refugees living in urban areas, but only secondary and tertiary care for refugees living in rural areas (UNHCR n.d.-b). UNHCR partially fills this gap by providing essential healthcare services for registered refugees in rural settings (UNHCR n.d.-b). Antenatal care provision by UNHCR is estimated to exceed 85% among registered refugees (UNHCR Pakistan 2024). Additionally, various local NGOs aim to bridge gaps in SRH care for unregistered refugees (Women's Refugee Commission 2016; International Planned Parenthood Federation 2023; UNFPA 2023; Raheel et al. 2012).

2.4 Stigma and Other Barriers to SHS Accessibility in MENA

2.4.1 Sexual Health Stigma in MENA

Sexual health stigma is a major barrier to accessing HIV and STI prevention and treatment throughout the MENA region. Punitive laws criminalizing same-sex relationships, sex work, and injection drug use, as well as legislation restricting the human rights of refugees, may exacerbate intersecting forms of sexual health stigma and disproportionately impact marginalized communities at greatest risk of STI transmission, including MSM, transgender women, and sex workers (Tohme et al. 2016a; Ballouz et al. 2020; Mumtaz et al. 2022; Tohme et al. 2016b; Aunon et al. 2015; Clark et al. 2017; Kaplan et al. 2015). Out of the 24 MENA countries, 21 have punitive laws against sex work, 19 have punitive laws against same-sex sex including death penalty in 7 of the countries, and 9 have laws prohibiting the possession of drugs for personal use (UNAIDS 2021).

HIV stigma has been repeatedly shown to be inversely correlated with HIV knowledge throughout multiple countries in the region, including Saudi Arabia, Lebanon, Yemen, and Jordan (Badahdah 2010; Youssef et al. 2021; Al Serouri et al. 2010). Evidence on the association between religiosity and HIV stigma in the region is conflicting and may be mediated by social factors including gender and education (Badahdah 2010; Youssef et al. 2021). HIV stigma is similarly prevalent among healthcare providers in MENA, primarily in the context of knowledge gaps related to transmission (Ballouz et al. 2020), and may be a modifiable risk factor to improving sexual health in the region. In Egypt, for instance, studies have demonstrated that healthcare workers are fearful of nosocomial HIV infection and may refuse to provide care to PLWH in the context of pervasive HIV stigma, limited exposure to PLWH, and insufficient institutional support (Kabbash et al. 2018; Aziz et al. 2023). Similarly in Jordan, healthcare workers caring for PLWH receive minimal formal HIV training and demonstrate low knowledge of HIV transmission as well as stigmatizing attitudes toward individuals who contracted the virus through sexual-risk behaviour (Saad et al. 2024).

HIV stigma may be a significant deterrent to seeking HIV testing and treatment among key populations, who may have related concerns of confidentiality violations (Ballouz et al. 2020). Qualitative studies among diverse populations in Lebanon, including cis-gender female sex workers, transgender women, and MSM, have identified concerns related to confidentiality of HIV testing and associated social and economic consequences as major barriers to HIV testing (Aunon et al. 2015; Clark et al. 2017; Kaplan et al. 2015).

2.4.2 Impact of Armed Conflict on SHS Accessibility

Additional barriers to accessing SHS in MENA are described in the context of destabilized health systems following decades of protracted armed conflict and massive forced displacement. While there is evidence from global humanitarian contexts that emergency-related disruptions to care may not significantly alter long-term ART accessibility (Casey 2015), such studies were conducted in settings with more robust public health infrastructure and during relatively transient crises, and thereby may not apply to MENA.

Indeed, the overburdening—and in some instances deliberate destruction—of already-fragile health systems in conflict settings may limit accessibility to ART (Mills et al. 2006). These findings were affirmed by a recent global systematic review, which identified a higher incidence of HIV in armed conflict and forced displacement settings due to disruptions in and reduced capacity of SHS availability (Marou et al. 2024). In Libya, for instance, where an association between war-related stress and injection drug use has been demonstrated (Elamouri et al. 2018), ongoing conflict and massive internal displacement have led to the disruption of SHS and greater geographic distribution of new HIV infections, potentially due to diminished access and adherence to ART (Daw et al. 2022). Similarly, in Syria, public health authorities described a 99% reduction in HIV surveillance among key populations since the civil war began, and significant decline in national voluntary counselling and testing (VCT) capacity (Khamis and Ghaddar 2018). Similar conflict-related impact on testing and surveillance has been described in Yemen (Country Progress Report 2013 Yemen 2013), while in Lebanon, an unprecedented economic crisis in the setting of prolonged political instability has forced the majority of VCT centres to close (Nabulsi et al. 2021; El-Jardali and El Bawab 2015).

Additionally, sexual health stigma may manifest with overt violence in armed conflict settings. In Yemen, for instance, there are reports of security forces preventing clinicians from providing care to PLWH due to pervasive stigmatization and misconceptions about transmission (Bashir et al. 2019).

2.4.3 Barriers to SHS Accessibility Among Forcibly Displaced Populations

Refugees' lived experiences of sexual health in MENA are characterized by different forms of stigma. Among Syrian refugee women, the largest population of forcibly displaced women globally (UNHCR 2023), sexual health stigma has been cited as a major barrier to healthcare accessibility in multiple countries with large refugee populations, including Jordan, Lebanon, and Turkey (Samari 2017). While Syrian refugee women in MENA have a high burden of unmet sexual and reproductive health needs, including reproductive tract infections, they face significant social limitations to seeking care. These limitations include sequelae of sexual and gender-based violence, adolescent pregnancy and menstrual irregularities, sexual health stigma, fears of mistreatment by healthcare workers, and a paucity of similar-gendered clinicians (Samari 2017; Reese Masterson et al. 2014). The impact of sexual health stigma on SHS accessibility has similarly been described among Syrian refugees resettled in high-income countries (Ussher et al. 2017), suggesting that this internalized stigma may be rooted in cultural norms and values which persist even following migration outside MENA.

Furthermore, the sequelae of untreated STIs may also be stigmatizing for women. For instance, infertility in MENA is gendered and has potentially devastating psychosocial consequences for women, whose social status is often linked with their ability to bear children (Serour 2008). Infertility is further stigmatized in Islamic settings due to religious doctrines that preclude adoption or use of certain assisted reproductive technologies (Abu-Rabia 2013).

Refugee MSM, transgender women, and other forcibly displaced key populations in MENA experience intersectional barriers to SHS accessibility, with multiple forms of stigma impeding care. For instance, Syrian refugee MSM in Lebanon, a high-risk population characterized by a high prevalence of sex work and condomless receptive anal intercourse (Tohme et al. 2016b), dually experience stigma on the basis of their sexual orientation and refugee status, the latter of which is associated with sexual-risk behaviour and poorer access to SHS (Tohme et al. 2016a). A comparative study of Syrian refugee and Lebanese host community MSM found that refugees experienced higher levels of both internalized and experienced MSM stigma, and were significantly less likely to report a lifetime history of HIV testing (Orr et al. 2022). In addition to limitations on SHS, stigma-related stressors have been shown to disproportionately impact the mental health of Syrian refugee MSM, who are more likely than their Lebanese counterparts to meet criteria for depression, anxiety, and post-traumatic stress disorder (Clark et al. 2021).

2.5 Conclusion

In conclusion, a multifaceted approach to improving HIV and STI prevention in MENA is urgently needed, as the current public health response remains inadequate to meet the evolving disease burden and sexual health needs of affected populations, including the large forcibly displaced population. The region faces unique challenges including conservative societal norms, fragmented health systems, the consequences of prolonged conflict and forced displacement, and pervasive stigma around sexuality and sexual health.

Efforts to improve sexual health outcomes must prioritize the expansion and integration of comprehensive SHS into primary healthcare systems, and strengthening partnerships with community-based organizations. These approaches have been proven effective in reaching marginalized populations, particularly in contexts where governmental responses are limited or constrained (Abu-Raddad et al. 2010c).

Additionally, addressing sexual health stigma and dismantling punitive laws and social barriers that impede access to care are essential steps toward achieving equitable and inclusive SHS. Effective strategies to mitigate sexual health stigma in particular are urgently needed across the region. For example, increasing HIV/STI training in undergraduate and graduate medical education programs and mandating HIV/STI stigma awareness activities among healthcare practitioners will help alleviate stigma within health care settings. Integrating SHS into well-established primary care settings, such as family planning programs, may also enhance accessibility and diminish stigma. Additionally, there is a need to develop and enact clear clinical standard practices to guide healthcare workers providing care for PLHIV and those affected by STIs in the region. Finally, sexual health models of care must be tailored to the health needs, cultural backgrounds, and living conditions of forcibly displaced populations in the region to ensure that no one is left behind.

References

Abi Zaki S et al (2020) Sexual practices, contraception methods, and self-reported urogenital symptoms among 116 refugee women in Beirut Lebanon. In: International AIDS conference

Abu-Rabia A (2013) Infertility and surrogacy in Islamic society: Socio-cultural, psychological, ethical, and religious dilemmas. Open Psychol J 6(1):54

Abu-Raddad LJ et al (2010a) Characterizing the HIV/AIDS epidemic in the Middle East and North Africa: Time for Strategic Action, Middle East and North Africa HIV/AIDS Epidemiology Synthesis Project. World Bank/UNAIDS/WHO Publication. The World Bank Press, Washington, DC

Abu-Raddad LJ et al (2010b) Epidemiology of HIV infection in the Middle East and North Africa. AIDS 24(Suppl 2):S5–S23

Abu-Raddad L et al (2010c) Characterizing the HIV/AIDS epidemic in the Middle East and North Africa: Time for Strategic Action. Middle East and North Africa HIV/AIDS Epidemiology Synthesis Project, World Bank/UNAIDS/WHO Publication. The World Bank Press, Washington, DC. Found at http://www-wds.worldbank.org/external/default/WDSContentServer/WDSP/IB/2010/06/04/000333038_20100604011533/Rendered/PDF/548890PUB0EPI11C10Dislosed061312010.pdf, Accessed 7 June 2023

Abu-Raddad LJ et al (2013) HIV and other sexually transmitted infection research in the Middle East and North Africa: promising progress? Sex Transm Infect 89(Suppl 3):iii1–iii4

Al Serouri A et al (2010) AIDS awareness and attitudes among Yemeni young people living in high-risk areas. EMHJ-Eastern Mediterr Health J 16(3):242–250

APIS Health Consulting Group (2016) Syrian Refugees crisis: impact on lebanese public hospitals. Available at: https://www.moph.gov.lb/DynamicPages/download_file/1396. Accessed 2 May 2024

Aunon FM et al (2015) An exploratory study of hiv risk behaviors and testing among male sex workers in Beirut, Lebanon. Soc Work Public Health 30(4):373–384

Aziz MM, Abdelrheem SS, Mohammed HM (2023) Stigma and discrimination against people living with HIV by health care providers in Egypt. BMC Health Serv Res 23(1):663

Badahdah AM (2010) Stigmatization of persons with HIV/AIDS in Saudi Arabia. J Transcult Nurs 21(4):386–392
Ballouz T, Gebara N, Rizk N (2020) HIV-related stigma among health-care workers in the MENA region. Lancet HIV 7(5):e311–e313
Bartels S, Hamill K (2014) Running out of time: Survival of Syrian refugee children in Lebanon. The FXB Center for Health and Human Rights at Harvard University
Bartels SA et al (2018) Making sense of child, early and forced marriage among Syrian refugee girls: a mixed methods study in Lebanon. BMJ Glob Health 3(1):e000509
Bashir F et al (2019) The realities of HIV prevention. A closer look at facilitators and challenges faced by HIV prevention programmes in Sudan and Yemen. Glob Health Action 12(1):1659098
Casey SE (2015) Evaluations of reproductive health programs in humanitarian settings: a systematic review. Confl Heal 9(1):1–14
Charles L, Denman K (2013) Syrian and palestinian Syrian refugees in Lebanon: The plight of women and children. J Int Women's Stud 14(5):96–111
Chemaitelly H et al (2019a) Epidemiology of Treponema pallidum, Chlamydia trachomatis, Neisseria gonorrhoeae, Trichomonas vaginalis, and herpes simplex virus type 2 among female sex workers in the Middle East and North Africa: systematic review and meta-analytics. J Glob Health 9(2):020408
Chemaitelly H et al (2019b) HIV epidemiology among female sex workers and their clients in the Middle East and North Africa: systematic review, meta-analyses, and meta-regressions. BMC Med 17(1):119
Chemaitelly H et al (2021) Global epidemiology of Neisseria gonorrhoeae in infertile populations: systematic review, meta-analysis and metaregression. Sex Transm Infect 97(2):157–169
Clark KA et al (2017) A qualitative analysis of multi-level barriers to HIV testing among women in Lebanon. Cult Health Sex 19(9):996–1010
Clark K et al (2021) Stigma, displacement stressors and psychiatric morbidity among displaced Syrian men who have sex with men (MSM) and transgender women: a cross-sectional study in Lebanon. BMJ Open 11(5):e046996
Country Progress Report 2013 Yemen (2013) National AIDS Program: Yemen
Dargham SR et al (2018) Herpes simplex virus type 2 seroprevalence among different national populations of Middle East and North African men. Sex Transm Dis 45(7):482–487
Daw MA, El-Bouzedi AH, Ahmed MO (2022) The impact of armed conflict on the prevalence and transmission dynamics of HIV infection in Libya. Front Public Health 10:779778
Dietrich W et al (2010) Multiple site sampling does not increase the sensitivity of Chlamydia trachomatis detection in infertility patients. Fertil Steril 93(1):68–71
Eggert-Kruse W et al (1996) Antibodies to chlamydia trachomatis in semen and relationship with parameters of male fertility. Hum Reprod 11(7):1408–1417
Eggert-Kruse W, Weltin M, Strowitzki T (2011) Are chlamydial lipopolysaccharide-directed antibodies in seminal plasma or serum clinically significant during investigation of male infertility? Urology 77(5):1101–1106
Elamouri FM et al (2018) "Now drugs in Libya are much cheaper than food": a qualitative study on substance use among young Libyans in post-revolution Tripoli. Libya Int J Drug Policy 53:23–31
El-Jardali F, El Bawab L (2015) K2P policy brief: addressing limitations to equitable access to healthcare services for people living with HIV in Lebanon. Knowledge to Policy (K2P) Center, Beirut
Fahme SA, Sieverding M, Abdulrahim S (2021) Sexual and reproductive health of adolescent Syrian refugee girls in Lebanon: a qualitative study of healthcare provider and educator perspectives. Reprod Health 18(1):113
Fahme SA et al (2024) Sexually transmitted infections among pregnant Syrian refugee women seeking antenatal care in Lebanon. J Travel Med 31:taae058
Fawaz M, Harb M, Al-Hage C (2021) Spatial patterns, gray spacing, and planning policy implications: the urbanization of forced population displacement in Lebanon. In: Urban recovery. Routledge, pp 65–89
Gluck C (2023) Forced returns from Pakistan deepen Afghanistan's humanitarian crisis [cited 2024 15 April]; Available from: https://www.unhcr.org/news/forced-returns-pakistan-deepen-afghanistan-s-humanitarian-crisis
Guterres A, Spiegel P (2012) The state of the world's refugees: adapting health responses to urban environments. JAMA 308(7):673–674
Hankins CA et al (2002) Transmission and prevention of HIV and sexually transmitted infections in war settings: implications for current and future armed conflicts. AIDS 16(17):2245–2252
Harfouche M et al (2023) Epidemiology of herpes simplex virus type 2 in the Middle East and North Africa: Systematic review, meta-analyses, and meta-regressions. J Med Virol 95(3):e28603
Heydari A et al (2016) Afghan refugees' experience of Iran's health service delivery. Int J Hum Rights Healthc 9(2):75–85
International Planned Parenthood Federation (2023) Empowering Afghan Refugees through Medical Camps in Pakistan [cited 2024 15 April]
Jauhiainen J, Eyvazlu D (2018) Urbanization, refugees and irregular migrants in Iran, 2017. In: Turun yliopiston maantieteen ja geologian laitoksen julkaisuja, p 9
Kabakian-Khasholian T et al (2020) Integration of sexual and reproductive health services in the provision of primary health care in the Arab States: status and a way forward. Sex Reprod Health Matters 28(2):1773693
Kabbash IA et al (2018) HIV/AIDS-related stigma and discrimination among health care workers at Tanta

University Hospitals, Egypt. Environ Sci Pollut Res Int 25:30755–30762
Kaplan RL et al (2015) Forms of safety and their impact on health: an exploration of HIV/AIDS-related risk and resilience among trans women in Lebanon. Health Care Women Int 36(8):917–935
Khamis J, Ghaddar A (2018) HIV/AIDS in Syria and the response of the National AIDS Program during the war. Sex Transm Infect 94(3):173–173
Khanani MR et al (2010) Concentrated epidemics of HIV, HCV, and HBV among Afghan refugees. J Infect 61(5):434–437
Lebanon: Refugees at risk in Covid-19 response (2020) Human Rights Watch
Marou V et al (2024) The impact of conflict on infectious disease: a systematic literature review. Confl Heal 18(1):27
McCall SJ et al (2023) Maternal and infant outcomes of Syrian and Palestinian refugees, Lebanese and migrant women giving birth in a tertiary public hospital in Lebanon: a secondary analysis of an obstetric database. BMJ Open 13(2):e064859
Mills EJ et al (2006) The impact of conflict on HIV/AIDS in sub-Saharan Africa. Int J STD AIDS 17(11):713–717
Miron ND et al (2013) Bacteriological agents which play a role in the development of infertility. Acta Microbiol Immunol Hung 60(1):41–53
Mohseni M et al (2023) Factors affecting the providing of sexual health services by midwives: a qualitative research in Iran. Iran J Nurs Midwifery Res 28(1):47–52
Mumtaz G et al (2010) Are HIV epidemics among men who have sex with men emerging in the Middle East and North Africa?: a systematic review and data synthesis. PLoS Med 8(8):e1000444
Mumtaz GR et al (2014a) HIV among people who inject drugs in the Middle East and North Africa: systematic review and data synthesis. PLoS Med 11(6):e1001663
Mumtaz GR, Riedner G, Abu-Raddad LJ (2014b) The emerging face of the HIV epidemic in the Middle East and North Africa. Curr Opin HIV AIDS 9(2):183–191
Mumtaz GR et al (2018) HIV incidence among people who inject drugs in the Middle East and North Africa: mathematical modelling analysis. J Int AIDS Soc 21(3):e25102
Mumtaz GR et al (2022) Status of the HIV epidemic in key populations in the Middle East and north Africa: knowns and unknowns. Lancet HIV 9(7):e506–e516
Nabulsi D et al (2021) Minimum initial service package (MISP) for sexual and reproductive health for women in a displacement setting: a narrative review on the Syrian refugee crisis in Lebanon. Reprod Health 18(1):58
Orr LV et al (2022) Sociodemographic characteristics and HIV risk behaviors of native-born and displaced Syrian men and transgender women who have sex with men in Lebanon. AIDS Behav 26(12):4004–4011
Panchenko S et al (2024) Sexual health challenges in migrant, immigrant, and displaced populations 2022–2023. Curr Opin Infect Dis 37(1):46–52
Population Reference Bureau (2024) 2023 World population data sheet. Available at: https://2023-wpds.prb.org/. Accessed 13 Apr 2024
Raheel H et al (2012) Knowledge, attitudes and practices of Contraception among Afghan Refugee women in Pakistan: a cross-sectional study. PLoS One 7(11):e48760
Reese Masterson A et al (2014) Assessment of reproductive health and violence against women among displaced Syrians in Lebanon. BMC Womens Health 14(1):25
Rostamkhani F et al (2015) Addressing the sexual problems of Iranian women in a primary health care setting: A quasi-experimental study. Iran J Nurs Midwifery Res 20(1):139–146
Saad RK et al (2024) HIV-related knowledge, attitude, practices, and stigma among healthcare providers caring for HIV in Jordan: identification of several organizational challenges. Heliyon 10(2):e24423
Saba HF et al (2013) Characterising the progress in HIV/AIDS research in the Middle East and North Africa. Sex Transm Infect 89(Suppl 3):iii5-9
Samari G (2017) Syrian refugee women's health in Lebanon, Turkey, and Jordan and recommendations for improved practice. World Med Health Policy 9(2):255–274
Serour G (2008) Medical and socio-cultural aspects of infertility in the Middle East. ESHRE Monogr 2008(1):34–41
Smolak A et al (2019) Epidemiology of Chlamydia trachomatis in the Middle East and north Africa: a systematic review, meta-analysis, and meta-regression. Lancet Glob Health 7(9):e1197–e1225
Starrs AM et al (2018) Accelerate progress-sexual and reproductive health and rights for all: report of the Guttmacher-Lancet Commission. Lancet 391(10140):2642–2692
Taylor MM et al (2022) Assessment of country implementation of the WHO global health sector strategy on sexually transmitted infections (2016-2021). PLoS One 17(5):e0263550
Tohme J et al (2016a) Psycho-social correlates of condom use and HIV testing among MSM refugees in Beirut, Lebanon. AIDS Behav 20(Suppl 3):417–425
Tohme J et al (2016b) HIV prevalence and demographic determinants of unprotected anal sex and HIV testing among male refugees who have sex with men in Beirut, Lebanon. AIDS Behav 20(3):408–416
Trafficking in Persons Report (2017) T.U.S.D.o. State, Editor. 2017, The United States Department of State
UNAIDS (2021) Global AIDS update: confronting inequalities – lessons for pandemic responses from 40 years of AIDS. Available from: https://www.unaids.org/en/resources/documents/2021/2021-global-aids-update Accessed 27 Nov 2021
UNAIDS (2023a) The path that ends AIDS: UNAIDS Global AIDS Update 2023. Available at: https://thepath.unaids.org/wp-content/themes/unaids2023/assets/files/2023_report.pdf. Accessed 14 Apr 2024

UNAIDS (2023b) Laws and Policies Analytics. Available: https://lawsandpolicies.unaids.org/. Accessed 8 Nov 2023

UNAIDS, AIDSinfo: Global Data on HIV Epidemiology and Response. Available at: https://aidsinfo.unaids.org/. Accessed 1 May 2024

UNFPA (2023) Ensuring care and safety for Afghan Women Refugees. Available from: https://pakistan.unfpa.org/en/news/ensuring-care-and-safety-afghan-women-refugees

UNHCR (2023) Global trends – Forced displacement in 2022. Geneva, Switzerland. Available at: https://www.unhcr.org/global-trends-report-2022. Accessed 13 Apr 2024

UNHCR (n.d.-a) Islamic Republic of Iran. Available at https://www.unhcr.org/countries/islamic-republic-iran. Accessed 2 May 2024

UNHCR (n.d.-b) Health Sector Strategy For Afghan Refugees Living in Pakistan 2014–2018. Available at: https://adsp.ngo/wp-content/uploads/2018/12/PS-6_Health-Sector-Strategy-For-Afghan-Refugees-Living-in-Pakistan-2014-2018.pdf. Accessed 2 May 2024

UNHCR Pakistan., Available at: https://www.unhcr.org/pk/health. Accessed 2 May 2024

UNRWA, Health Services Provided by UNRWA. Available at https://www.unrwa.org/what-we-do/services?program=39. Accessed 1 May 2024

Ussher JM et al (2017) Negotiating discourses of shame, secrecy, and silence: Migrant and Refugee Women's experiences of sexual embodiment. Arch Sex Behav 46(7):1901–1921

Vaccarella S, Bruni L, Seoud M (2013) Burden of human papillomavirus infections and related diseases in the extended Middle East and North Africa region. Vaccine 31(Suppl 6):G32–G44

Women's Refugee Commission (2016) Building national resilience for sexual and reproductive health: learning from current experiences

World Health Organization (2023) Epidemiological fact sheet: HIV statistics, globally and by WHO region, 2023. Available at: https://cdn.who.int/media/docs/default-source/hq-hiv-hepatitis-and-stis-library/j0294-who-hiv-epi-factsheet-v7.pdf?sfvrsn=5cbb3393_7. Accessed 21 Apr 2024

World Health Organization (2024a) Regional Office for the Eastern Mediterranean, Understanding the epidemiological landscape of sexually transmitted infections in the World Health Organization Eastern Mediterranean Region: Implications for strategic action. Eastern Mediterranean Sexually Transmitted Infections Epidemiology Synthesis Project. World Health Organization. Regional Office for the Eastern Mediterranean

World Health Organization (2024b) HPV Dashboard. Available at: https://www.who.int/teams/immunization-vaccines-and-biologicals/diseases/human-papillomavirus-vaccines-(HPV)/hpv-clearing-house/hpv-dashboard. Accessed 1 May 2024

Yasmine R, Moughalian C (2016) Systemic violence against Syrian refugee women and the myth of effective intrapersonal interventions. Reprod Health Matters 24(47):27–35

Yassin N (2018) 101 facts & figures on the Syrian refugee crisis. Issam Fares Institute for Public Policy and International Affairs, American University of Beirut, Beyrut, pp 2017–2018

Youssef L et al (2021) Knowledge, attitudes and practices towards people living with HIV/AIDS in Lebanon. PLoS One 16(3):e0249025

Zakian Khorramabadi F et al (2023) Access to health care for Afghan immigrants and refugees: an ethico-legal analysis based on the Iranian health law system. J Med Ethics Hist Med 16:12

3 Cervical Cancer Prevention Among Refugees and Displaced Persons: New Opportunities to Reach the Underserved

Karel Blondeel Bombeke, Mathilde Forestier, Mariluz Hernandez, Dur-e-Nayab Waheed, Felix Ricardo Burdier Custodio, Isotta Rossoni, Valeska Padovese, and Maribel Almonte

Contents

K. B. Bombeke (✉)
Department of Noncommunicable Diseases, World Health Organization, Geneva, Switzerland

Faculty of Medicine and Health Sciences, Ghent University, Ghent, Belgium
e-mail: karel@researchersconsultants.com

M. Forestier · M. Hernandez · M. Almonte
Department of Noncommunicable Diseases, World Health Organization, Geneva, Switzerland
e-mail: forestierm@who.int; hernandezmari@who.int; almontem@who.int

Dur-e-Nayab Waheed · F. R. Burdier Custodio
Centre for Evaluation of Vaccination, University of Antwerp, Antwerp, Belgium
e-mail: nayab.waheed@uantwerpen.be; ricardo.burdier@uantwerpen.be

I. Rossoni
Van Vollenhoven Institute -Leiden Law School, Leiden University, Leiden, The Netherlands

V. Padovese
Bridges2Health&Rights NGO, Msida, Malta

Genitourinary Clinic, Department of Dermatology and Venereology, Mater Dei Hospital, Msida, Malta
e-mail: valeska.padovese@gov.mt

V. Padovese, I. Rossoni (eds.), *Intersections of Sexual Health, Migration and Sexualised Violence*, Sustainable Development Goals Series, https://doi.org/10.1007/978-3-032-20707-4_3

Abstract

This chapter presents the literature and available data on cervical cancer prevention coverage, barriers, and opportunities among refugees and other displaced populations. It presents updated WHO guidelines and innovations, both technological and interventional, which hold promise for reaching underserved women and individuals with a cervix. Finally, using a socio-ecological model, the chapter identifies and analyzes personal, interpersonal (related to healthcare providers), organizational (healthcare facilities), structural (health systems), and contextual (cultural, religious, environmental, etc.) barriers to vaccination and screening, as well as related facilitating measures and opportunities.

Keywords

HPV · Cervical cancer · Migration · Prevention · Vaccination · Screening

3.1 Introduction

While cervical cancer is a preventable disease, it is the fourth most common cancer in women and individuals with a cervix[1] worldwide, with over 660,000 new cases and almost 350,000 cervical cancer deaths in 2022, of which an estimated 94% in low- and middle-income countries (LMICs) (Cancer Today 2024). The global number of deaths per year is projected to increase to 416,000 in 2035 if no action is taken to improve prevention (Fig. 3.1).

Cervical cancer is the most common type of cancer in 25 countries and the leading cause of cancer death in 37 countries, mainly in sub-Saharan Africa, South America, and South-Eastern Asia (Bray et al. 2024). Maternal deaths from cervical cancer were responsible for a fifth of an estimated 1,047,000 children that became maternal orphans in 2020 due to cancer (Guida et al. 2022).

Ninety-five percent of cervical cancer cases are caused by persistent cervical human papillomavirus (HPV) infection (Cervical cancer 2025). Typically, it takes 15–20 years for abnormal cervical cells to progress to cancer, but in women with weakened immune systems, such as untreated HIV, this process can be faster and take 5–10 years (Cervical cancer 2025). Cervical cancer deaths can be prevented by primary, secondary, and tertiary prevention interventions: (1) vaccinating against HPV infection; (2) screening to detect cervical pre-cancerous lesions, which can be treated to prevent progression to cervical cancer; (3) early detection followed by prompt treatment to cure cervical cancer (Cervical cancer 2025).

[1]This chapter refers to "women and individuals with a cervix" as a population, as cervical cancer screening and treatment should be provided to cisgender women and transgender men, non-binary and intersex individuals who have a cervix. We did not find any specific data on cervical cancer screening and treatment for these populations who are refugees or forcibly displaced. Health care research and systems in itself, including screening and treatment services for cervical pre-cancer and cancer, need to be more inclusive of transgender, intersex, and non-binary persons.

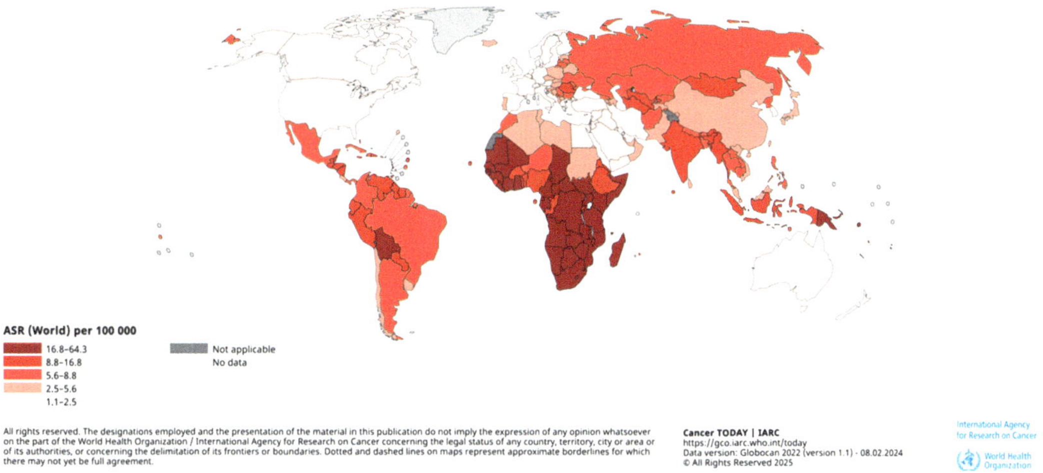

Fig. 3.1 Age-standardized cervical cancer mortality rate per 100,000 women in 2022. (Reproduced with permission from IARC/WHO, generated by data visualization app on IARC https://gco.iarc.fr/today/en/dataviz)

The regional differences in cervical cancer burden are related to both inequalities in access to vaccination, screening and treatment services, risk factors such as HIV infection, and social and economic determinants such as sex and gender biases and poverty.

The UN Refugee Agency (UNHCR) reported 122.6 million forcibly displaced persons[2] by mid 2024, of which more than half were internally displaced (https://www.unhcr.org/external/component/header 2025). Even though some of the top ten countries of origin of refugees and other displaced populations have relatively low cervical cancer mortality rates (typically in the Middle Eastern region), in other countries, such as the Democratic Republic of the Congo, Somalia, or Venezuela, mortality rates are high.[3]

Refugee and other displaced women and individuals with a cervix have often been confronted with conflict, (sexual) violence, or persecution in their countries of origin, decreasing their access sometimes to already fragile healthcare services. As such, both the context resulting in their displacement and the new context after displacement may increase risk factors for cervical cancer (among others STIs, including HIV), worsen social and economic determinants, and deprive refugee and other displaced women of prevention, potentially leading to cervical cancer burden disparities (Pannetier et al. 2018).

Data on cervical cancer-related mortality and disability among refugee and other displaced women and individuals with a cervix is scarce, as well as data on the comparison of burden with the host population or the evolution of burden inequalities over time. Robust data on cancer incidence and mortality in humanitarian and conflict-affected settings may be challenging to obtain due to non-existing or disrupted health information systems and cancer registries and, if national health datasets do exist, refugee and migrant health-related variables are not commonly included (Casolino et al. 2025; World report on the health of refugees and migrants 2024). Higher cancer mortality rates have been observed in

[2]Forcibly displaced people encompasses refugees, asylum-seekers, other people in need of international protection, and internally displaced people. It includes refugees and other displaced people not covered by UNHCR's mandate and excludes other categories such as returnees and non-displaced stateless people.

[3]In 2024, these countries were Syrian Arab Republic, Sudan, Afghanistan, Ukraine, Democratic Republic of the Congo, Venezuela, State of Palestine, Colombia, Somalia, and Yemen.

humanitarian and conflict-affected settings compared with more stable settings (Casolino et al. 2025). Additionally, and contrary to other cancers, the risk for cervical cancer also seems to be higher among refugee women in stable settings across the European region (WHO), compared to the host populations, and they are more likely to be diagnosed at a later stage in the disease (Report on the health of refugees 2018).

In this chapter, we present the literature and available data on cervical cancer prevention coverage, barriers, and opportunities among refugees and other displaced populations. Moreover, we will present the updated WHO guidelines and innovations, both technological and interventional, which hold promise for reaching underserved women and individuals with a cervix. While there are many different obstacles in the various settings, successful implementation seems feasible.

3.2 Cancer Elimination and Cancer Care Initiatives

Boosting the World Health Organization's (WHO) earlier work on guidance on cervical cancer prevention, the Director General called to action to eliminate cervical cancer as a public health problem and subsequently launched the Cervical Cancer Elimination Initiative (CCEI). The Initiative developed the Global Strategy for cervical cancer elimination, setting the threshold to reach elimination at the age-adjusted rate of four invasive cervical cancers per 100,000 women a year (Global strategy to accelerate the elimination 2025). Three targets were set for countries to be reached by 2030 to be in the path toward elimination:

- 90% of girls to be vaccinated fully against HPV by age 15
- 70% of women to be screened using a high-performance test by ages 35 and 45
- 90% of women identified with cervical disease to be receiving treatment and care

The strategy explicitly called for tailored approaches to resolve the health inequities that touch underserved populations, or those who live in vulnerable conditions.

While the majority of global cancer deaths occur in LMICs and is expected to rise, these countries also bear the highest number of humanitarian crises and host 71% of refugees worldwide, adding additional stress to their health systems (Bray et al. 2024; Casolino et al. 2025; UNHCR, the UN Refugee Agency 2025). As cancer care in general has been neglected in humanitarian responses, a high-level manifesto following the first Global Summit on War and Cancer in 2023 has called for cancer care to be established as a core pillar of an emergency response plan in all conflict settings and the inclusion of cancer in humanitarian settings into the political agendas of the United Nations (Ghebreyesus et al. 2024).

Specifically for cervical cancer, HPV vaccination has not usually been included in health guidance or programming for humanitarian responses and even less so screening and treatment of cervical precancer or cancer.

3.3 Vaccination, Screening, Treatment Coverage

3.3.1 Vaccination

In 2023, an estimated 27% of girls globally had received at least one HPV-vaccine dose, which is 10% more than in 2019, but still far from the strategy's 90% target (Fig. 3.2) (WHO Immunization Data portal – Global 2025). The lowest income countries are entitled to receive support by GAVI, The Vaccine Alliance, to implement HPV vaccination. In this group of countries, the overall coverage increased from 4% in

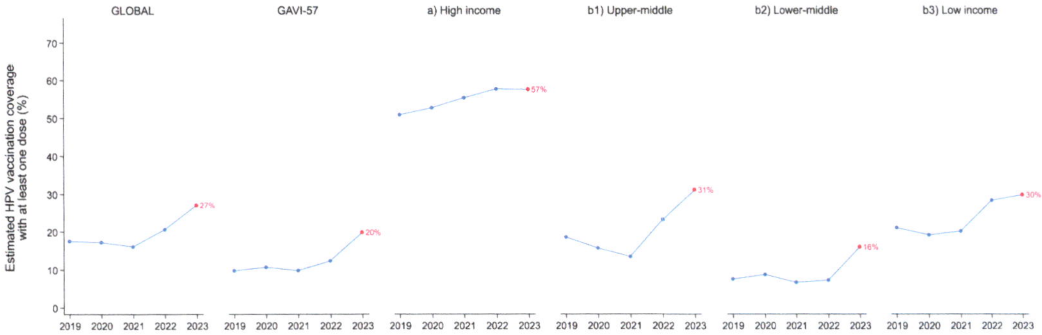

Fig. 3.2 Global estimates of HPV vaccine coverage in girls of ages 9-14y (at least one dose), by year. World Health Organization. WHO Immunization Data portal – Human Papillomavirus (HPV) vaccination coverage. Immunization Data. July 15, 2024. https://immunizationdata.who.int/global/wiise-detail-page/human-papillomavirus-(hpv)-vaccination-coverage-vaccination-coverage)

2019 to 16% in 2023 (Snapshot 2025). In general, coverage varies widely across countries grouped by income (World Bank).

Although vaccine introductions are increasing, coverage is suboptimal. In 2023, a quarter of the countries with implemented HPV vaccination programs had not yet reached a coverage of 50%, suggesting important implementation challenges and/or access barriers in these countries.

Refugees and other displaced persons face many barriers to be vaccinated against HPV due to the absence or disruption of vaccine systems in their countries, as well as personal, socio-structural, and physical conditions including their mobility. Vaccination programs in the host countries may also not be offering the HPV vaccine yet, as it has only been since 2009 that WHO has recommended the inclusion of HPV vaccination into national immunization programs, and only in countries where cervical cancer is a public health priority and where cost-effective and sustainable implementation of the vaccine is feasible (Knights et al. 2024; Organization WH 2016).

Of the top ten host countries, only Colombia and Ethiopia had national HPV-vaccination programs in place.[4] Contrary to Sudan where cervical cancer prevention, screening or early detection programs for the general population are lacking due to the instability of public health leadership and limited public financing. This leaves little space for vaccination in internally displaced and refugee populations (Husain et al. 2022).

Moreover, in humanitarian settings, young girls may lack birth certificates and may not be included in birth registries, increasing their chances of being missed in HPV-vaccination campaigns. This also complicates estimating vaccination coverage in these populations, due to the uncertainty regarding the denominator, i.e. the number of eligible girls.

3.3.2 Screening and Treatment

Although around four out of five countries globally report to have national cervical cancer screening (CCS) guidelines, in 2022, only an

[4] In 2024, these countries were Sudan, Syrian Arab Republic, Democratic Republic of the Congo, Colombia, Ethiopia, Yemen, Turkey, Afghanistan, Somalia, and the Islamic Republic of Iran.

Table 3.1 Estimated number of women ever screened by any type of screening and HPV test and screening coverage until 2022

	Screening ever in lifetime—by any type of screening				Screening ever in lifetime—by an HPV testing			
	Number of screened women in millions		Coverage		Number of screened women in millions		Coverage	
	N	(95% CI)	%	(95% CI)	N	(95% CI)	%	(95% CI)
World	407.1	(356.3–462.3)	38%	(33–43%)	84.6	(69.1–101.3)	7%	(7–10%)
Coverage by country income level								
High income	150.0	(131.5–170.1)	81%	(71–92%)	62.2	(48.5–77.5)	33%	(26–42%)
Low and middle income	257.1	(212.7–306.4)	29%	(24–35%)	22.3	(16.7–28.3)	2%	(2–3%)
Upper-middle income	215.2	(168.6–266.2)	52%	(40–64%)	22.0	(16.6–27.8)	5%	(4–7%)
Lower-middle income	33.1	(30.1–36.6)	8%	(7–9%)	0.25	(0.19–0.31)	<0.1%	(0–0%)
Low-income	8.8	(7.6–10.1)	12%	(10–14%)	0.09	(0.06–0.12)	<0.1%	(0–0%)

estimated 37% of women aged 30–49 years had been screened for cervical cancer with any method at least once in their lifetime. If HPV testing only is considered—the preferred screening method following WHO's most recent guidelines—a mere 8% of the target population is estimated to have been screened at least once in their life. Similar to HPV vaccination coverage, there are big differences between country groups, based on income level, as shown in Table 3.1, with HPV-based screening being hardly introduced in lower-middle and low-income countries.

In the top ten host countries, there are only three countries (Turkey, Colombia, and the Islamic Republic of Iran) where more than 20% of women between 30 and 49 years had been screened by any method (visual inspection with acetic acid, cervical cytology, HPV testing), at least once in the past 5 years. Limited data on CCS indicate coverage disparities between displaced populations and the host population. A systematic review from 2014 showed that only 25% of asylum seekers had undergone a cervical pap test compared with 62% in the host population, increasing the risk of being diagnosed with late stage disease, reducing the likelihood of effective treatment and management (Report on the health of refugees 2018; Hadgkiss and Renzaho 2014; World Health Organization 2014).

In the 2020 Survey for Health Care Needs Analysis of Syrian Population under Temporary Protection, 86.6% of Syrian refugee women between 15 and 49 stated not having been screened in Turkey (Turkey: MoH/SIHHAT 2025). A systematic review on the provision of sexual health services to internally displaced women and refugees in Africa did not find any study documenting CCS services, which may be showing the absence of both services and efforts to gather data on the use thereof (Ngwibete et al. 2024).

3.4 Barriers to Primary and Secondary Cervical Cancer Prevention for Refugee and Other Forcibly Displaced Persons

Most research on barriers to vaccination and screening has concentrated on migrant populations, or populations with a birth country other than the study country (not necessarily migrants), in high-income countries, sometimes including smaller populations of refugees. More specific populations such as undocumented migrants, transmigrants (in transit through a country on the way to a desired final destination country), or asylum seekers have also been included. Of the studies that do target refugee populations, very few are conducted in countries where the most refugees reside. In a recent systematic review on barriers to CCS among refugee women, only one included study was done in low- or middle-income settings (Hossain et al. 2025).

Barriers to healthcare and more specifically to cervical cancer prevention depend on different factors related to specific circumstances, including the type of settings these populations reside in (in/formal refugee camps, closed/open centers, or settled, urban/rural), or the health systems and the cervical cancer prevention policies and practices of both origin and host countries.

While these barriers may be stratified following different models, here we will present them following an adapted social ecological model, focusing on overarching or common traits on the personal, interpersonal (related to healthcare providers), organizational (healthcare facilities), structural (health systems), and contextual (cultural, religious, environmental, etc.) levels (McLeroy et al. 1988) (Fig. 3.3). These five levels overlap and interact, as personal level decisions may be influenced by culture or religion, or the work of healthcare providers may be impacted by decisions at the health policy level.

3.4.1 Personal

An often recurring barrier is the lack of awareness of and knowledge about HPV infection, the burden of cervical cancer, and how to prevent it (Haworth et al. 2014; Kim et al. 2017; Allen et al. 2019; Babatunde-Sowole et al. 2020; Zhang et al. 2017; Davidson et al. 2022; Ghebrendrias et al. 2021). An infection with carcinogenic HPV (cHPV) and even a prevalent precancerous lesion may stay unnoticed due to the lack of symptoms. Consequently, women and individuals with a cervix lacking awareness and knowledge may perceive themselves at low risk and not seek for or participate in cervical cancer prevention services (Kim et al. 2017; Marques et al. 2020; Parajuli et al. 2020). Lack of knowledge and misinformation may also lead to hesitancy to use health services, or complacency about the need for vaccination (Ensuring the integration 2025). Qualitative research in Turkish migrant communities has shown that women would attend screening services if they had been informed and invited (Altaş and Sezerol 2025).

Fear, shyness, or discomfort related to the procedure or negative anticipations about the results, which may partly be caused by a lack of knowledge or previous negative experiences, may have migrant and refugee women and individuals with a cervix to seek or postpone screening visits (Haworth et al. 2014; Ghebrendrias et al. 2021; Marques et al. 2020; Lor et al. 2018; Kue et al. 2017).

Language issues are one of the most commonly cited barriers among displaced and migrant populations alike. This may cause women and individuals with a cervix not to grasp information about vaccination and screening to prevent cervical cancer, but may also compromise their privacy when their relatives serve as interpreters, leaving women and individuals with a cervix uncomfortable to talk about intimate issues (Haworth et al. 2014; Ghebrendrias et al. 2021; Parajuli et al. 2020; Altaş and Sezerol 2025; Lor et al. 2018).

Lastly, the shorter the women and individuals with a cervix have stayed in a host country, the less the chance they have participated in screening; this has been partially explained by both a lack of knowledge about the country's health services and migration-related stress (Barrera-Castillo et al. 2020).

3.4.2 Interpersonal

A lack of perceived social support, by the partner, family, or friends, has been shown to have a negative impact on CCS participation (Barrera-Castillo et al. 2020).

Previous negative experiences with healthcare providers—such as among other things not being professional or friendly, no experience with migrant populations, pain, or bleeding—during

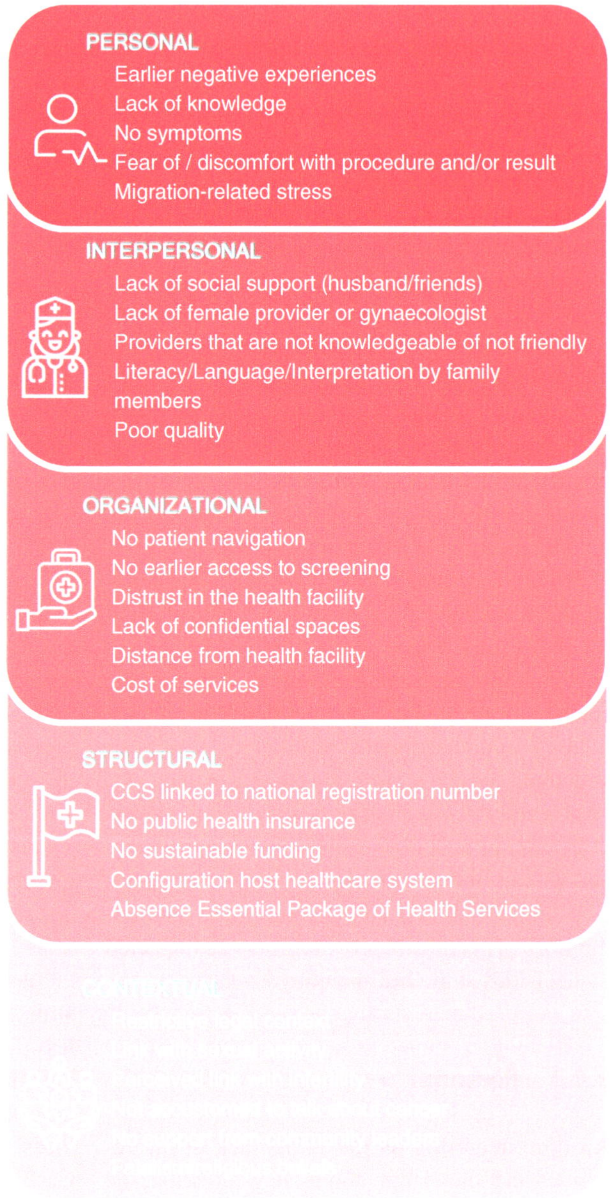

Fig. 3.3 Social ecological model presenting barriers to HPV vaccination and CCS for refugee and displaced women and individuals with a cervix

screening in the country of origin or host country, including in refugee camps, may prevent women and individuals with a cervix from trusting or using these services (Marques et al. 2020; Parajuli et al. 2020; Lor et al. 2018). Some studies also showed that a lack of a female healthcare provider or a gynecologist contributed to nonparticipation (Kim et al. 2017; Ghebrendrias et al. 2021; Marques et al. 2020).

3.4.3 Organizational

As has been mentioned above, in many of the countries of origin of refugee women and refugee individuals with a cervix, preventative health services, including HPV vaccination or CCS, are often not available or of limited quality (Davidson et al. 2022; Ghebrendrias et al. 2021). They may not be accustomed to these services or to attend regular medical checkups and hence be unaware of their cervical cancer prevention needs (Marques et al. 2020; Lor et al. 2018).

Refugee women and individuals with a cervix face practical barriers to access, such as not being able to reach healthcare facilities due to mobility restrictions, transport or road blockades, or limited availability of appointments and the need for childcare (Haworth et al. 2014; Abdullahi et al. 2009). Another practical barrier is the lack of availability of the refugee's health records, including vaccination cards and earlier screening results or treatments related to cervical cancer, often due to lack of synchronized data in a single platform (Cata-Preta et al. 2024).

3.4.4 Structural

As mentioned above, both host countries and those of origin, especially from LMICs, may lack cervical cancer services due to funding constraints. The vaccination and screening policies and practices of host country that do have the funds may still be a barrier to refugee women and individuals with a cervix when they are incongruent with their realities and needs. Host country policies not enabling catch up vaccination to eligible refugee girls and women and individuals with a cervix may lead to cancer burden inequalities for decades to come. Likewise, policies that do not include potential screening beyond the age of 65 years may be detrimental for refugee women and individuals with a cervix that have never been screened or have no history of a negative test. On the other side of the age spectrum, initiating screening regardless of sexual debut may anatomically not be possible in those refugee women and individuals with a cervix that have suffered infibulation (Walker et al. 2022).

Further, the configuration of the health system of the host country is an important barrier when screening programs are based on National Population Registers that include only legal residents or those being registered in the national health system (Azerkan et al. 2015; O'Donnell et al. 2016). For countries that have not included cervical cancer prevention in their essential health package, cost may be impeding girls from being vaccinated and women and individuals with a cervix from being screened (Haworth et al. 2014; Kim et al. 2017; Lor et al. 2018).

Related to the language barrier mentioned above, information about cervical cancer is frequently only provided in the host country's native language(s), preventing migrant women and individuals with a cervix to get properly informed about screening practices in the country. Refugee women also indicated that navigating the host country's health system can be confusing, resulting in either having difficulties to make appointments or missing appointments (Lor et al. 2018).

3.4.5 Contextual

Even though health is a fundamental human right for all, including for refugees and other displaced populations, national legislation may be a barrier to the entitlement of these populations to receive affordable and adequate care. Refugee women and individuals with a cervix may not want to be identified in and through health services out of fear to be expelled or incarcerated.

Next to the legal context, the cultural and religious context may also determine the beliefs about and attitudes toward cervical cancer prevention. Cultural notions concerning the sacred body or beliefs that cancer is a fatal disease may impede access to vaccination and screening for many women and individuals with a cervix (Kim et al. 2017; Parajuli et al. 2020; Abdullahi et al. 2009; Hamdiui et al. 2022). Talking about cancer or gynecologic issues is in some cultures a taboo (Ghebrendrias et al. 2021). Due to the connection with sexual health, some may be afraid to be judged when using the services or if having a positive screening result. In a culture where the preservation of fertility of girls and women is estimated to be of high value, there may be skepticism over health interventions concerning the female reproductive system (Hamdiui et al. 2022).

3.5 Facilitating Measures

Most of the barriers discussed seem to be similar to those that refugees face in accessing healthcare in general (Marques et al. 2020). Across the literature, measures are being suggested and have been implemented enabling access to cervical cancer prevention interventions for migrants and refugees, contributing to a migrant and refugee-friendly health system.

Cervical cancer prevention should start with providing women and individuals with a cervix with relevant and easy-to-understand information about sexual and reproductive health (SRH) in general, and cervical cancer specifically, in places they frequent, to increase awareness and prevent misinformation within the community or in on- and offline media channels (Ghebrendrias et al. 2021; Tazinya et al. 2023). when possible, men and boys should be engaged as allies and partners in achieving SRH goals, including cervical cancer (Aantjes and Govender 2024).

It is important that national cervical cancer prevention health policies include strategies to allow access to refugee and displaced populations and are properly adapted to their situation and needs (Altaş and Sezerol 2025). It has been suggested that primary healthcare has the potential to respond adequately and cost-effectively to cervical cancer health needs including for refugees (van Loenen et al. 2018; Troisi et al. 2025). One such example are the Migrant Health Centers, established within the framework of primary healthcare institutions, in regions in Turkey with significant refugee populations to improve access to preventive and primary healthcare services for Syrian refugees (Turkey: MoH/SIHHAT 2025). Additionally, Syrian cancer care professionals were employed to bridge language and cultural gaps, improving the integration and effectiveness of the services (Casolino et al. 2025).

Cervical cancer programs should be well promoted (for example, by written or verbal invitation) in relevant languages, should be easy to navigate, should have no costs associated, and should be adapted to the context. Implementation research on cervical cancer prevention in refugee and displaced populations is however close to non-existent.

Respectful, multilingual and knowledgeable, and in some contexts female-only, healthcare providers have been mentioned commonly as important facilitators for the delivery of cervical cancer prevention programs. Alternative delivery methods have been suggested, such as educational sessions by people trusted by women and individuals with a cervix and through community activities (Haworth et al. 2014; Lor et al. 2018; Allen et al. 2019). It is important to understand cultural differences about sexuality and gender or past traumatic personal experiences to elaborate strategies that can increase acceptance and positive attitudes toward the proposed prevention programs (Marques et al. 2020). A study showing that women who did not attend cervical screening did not consider themselves to be non-attenders seem to indicate that they were not a priori against cervical screening, while another study indicated that women were very open to screening and vaccination with the right messaging (Azerkan et al. 2015; Allen et al. 2019). This leaves a window of opportunities to increase vaccination and screening coverage.

In addition to identifying the needs of women and individuals with a cervix, it is essential for countries to understand and adapt service delivery models to different contexts. For example, service provision in humanitarian settings may differ significantly from delivery in urban or community-based settings for migrant populations. Equally important is mapping key stakeholders and understanding who shapes the narrative within these populations, as this can enhance both uptake and relevance of services. Service provision should be culturally safe and inclusive (Costa et al. 2024). Culturally sensitive community-based approaches tailored to individual ethnic groups within broader immigrant communities in the USA have proven successful in improving cancer screening uptake and showed evidence of reaching individuals who had never been screened. (Milenkov et al. 2020) Including discussions about religious values in relation to cervical cancer prevention facilitated by respected female mosque members have also been suggested (Hamdiui et al. 2022).

As refugee settlements are shifting from formal refugee camps to informal tent camps and urban-based decentralized settlement, other delivery methods should be considered. One such approach is a mobile clinic that provided sexual and gender-based violence care among Syrian refugees in Lebanon. Qualitative research has shown it is a promising approach that improves the well-being of refugee women and girls; in particular, the free and flexible service delivery in the women's own communities can mitigate access barriers related to transportation, checkpoints, cost, and gendered expectations around mobility and domestic responsibilities (Lilleston et al. 2018).

Mhealth is also increasingly being used to improve HPV vaccine and cancer screening uptake and seems to be an effective method that could be used in refugee and displaced populations to overcome among other things awareness, cultural, and language barriers (Ou et al. 2023; Schliemann et al. 2022). A Nepalese NGO is experimenting with a mobile application in twelve languages to increase vaccine uptake among migrant communities (Box 3.1).[5]

Box 3.1: Mass HPV Vaccination in Cox's Bazar Refugee Camps in Bangladesh (Strengthening Health Initiatives 2025)

Limited country examples exist on service delivery among hard-to-reach girls in low-resource settings. Bangladesh conducted a mass HPV vaccination campaign among forcibly displaced girls from Myanmar living in Cox's Bazar. The was the first of its kind conducted in a refugee setting, targeting over 63,000 girls aged 10–14, both in and out of school, across 33 camps. Vaccination was offered through 68 fixed healthcare, focusing on accessibility, safety, and coverage. Over 2000 personnel, including community health workers, supervisors, vaccinators, and managers were mobilized. Community engagement played a central role, as local leaders, including Majhis and Imams, helped build trust and sessions were targeting vaccine hesitancy in mothers. Misinformation was addressed by counter rumors and fears.

Registration was streamlined using existing ID systems managed by UNHCR. Real-time monitoring, flexible scheduling (five main campaign days and two mop-up days), and strong coordination allowed for rapid adjustments, leading to increased demand and 109.8% coverage, exceeding the original target.

Key lessons include the value of careful planning, local leadership engagement, responsive communication, and flexible delivery models. The campaign highlights how inclusive, community-driven strategies can succeed even in challenging humanitarian contexts.[6]

3.6 Opportunities

3.6.1 One-Dose Vaccination

In 2022, WHO advised the off-label use of a single dose instead of two-dose HPV vaccination in girls and boys between 9 and 20, and its efficacy is further being reconfirmed by ongoing research (Whitworth et al. 2024; Bassett et al. 2025; Human papillomavirus vaccines 2022). The one-dose option has already been adopted by 72 countries, of which 63 are LMICs (HPV Dashboard 2025). While one-dose vaccination

[5]Communication Pema Lhaki Lama, NFCC—Nepal during HPV Board Global Meeting: Cervical Cancer Prevention and Control in Displaced Populations, 13–14 February 2025, Istanbul, Turkey.

[6]Communication Muhibul Kashem, PATH - Bangladesh during the HPV Board Global Meeting: Cervical Cancer Prevention and Control in Displaced Populations, 13–14 February 2025, Istanbul, Turkey.

should facilitate and accelerate country introductions and increase coverage of existing programs, it also holds promise for the inclusion of refugee and displaced populations. With no need for a second dose, vaccination programs in this population may overcome the transiency challenges and loss to follow-up.

Even though there have been constraints on the vaccine supply side, it seems that it would meet demands as of 2026 (WHO HPV Vaccine Global Market Study 2022; Garland et al. 2024). In the near future, more low-income countries are planning introductions and they should seize this opportunity to close health disparities and include refugees and displaced population from the onset of the program. In Uganda, for example, the Refugee Health sector integrated planning has already included refugees in the one-dose vaccination scheme, and health data on refugees are being included in the DHS.[7]

3.6.2 Self-Collection of Samples and New HPV Tests for Screening

Since the 2021 guidelines for cervical cancer screening, WHO's preferred primary screening method is an HPV nucleic acid test (NAT), and it is suggested that samples for these tests can be taken by the provider or self-collected by the women and individuals with a cervix to be screened (World Health Organization 2021a; World Health Organization 2021b). Programs that offer HPV self-collection of samples have shown to increase participation; however, a qualitative study in migrants in the Netherlands has indicated that women may regard their ability to correctly perform self-sampling as low or expect a healthcare provider to take the sample (Hamdiui et al. 2022; Wong and Wong 2024). Increasing awareness about the quality of self-sampling and self-collection itself and the applying opt-out strategies should help to overcome these barriers.

Refugee and displaced women and individuals with a cervix often reside in conditions that are challenging them to follow up on results of tests or come back for treatments. HPV test that can be used at the point-of-care (POC), enabling the result within the same visit, could therefore be a game changer in cervical cancer screening if there is a capacity for immediate treatment of screen-positive women and individuals with a cervix. However, affordable HPV POC tests have yet to become available. Although the market is very active, with over 260 distinct commercial HPV tests (and over 500 test variants) in 2023, only around 20 of those meet internationally recognized clinical validation standards, and none of those seems to qualify as an affordable POC option for humanitarian settings (Poljak et al. 2024). Nonetheless, technological advances have enabled the potential for such tests and WHO has published target product profiles for HPV screening tests to detect cervical pre-cancer and cancer, one for tests used in the laboratory, and a separate one for tests to be used at the POC, motivating developers and manufacturers alike to direct their efforts to the global health needs (World Health Organization 2024).

3.6.3 Thermal Ablators for Pre-cancer Treatment

As mentioned above, increased screening is only ethically sound if treatment capacity is available to offer sufficient and quality treatments. In 2014, WHO has provided guidelines for the use of thermal ablation as first-line treatment for cervical pre-cancer lesions in eligible women and individuals with a cervix (World Health Organization 2019). A thermal ablator is a simple kind of equipment, is lightweight (can weigh less than 2 kg), and is easily portable. The treatment is based on short application(s) of a reusable metallic probe that is electrically heated to approximately 100 °C, leading to epithelial and stromal destruction. Like cryotherapy, thermal ablation can be provided by a variety of healthcare per-

[7] Communication Ronald Nyakoojo, UNHCR—Uganda during the HPV Board Global Meeting: Cervical Cancer Prevention and Control in Displaced Populations, 13–14 February 2025, Istanbul, Turkey.

sonnel, including primary healthcare workers, and is typically performed without anesthesia. The advantage of thermal ablation over cryotherapy is its portability as it can be powered by batteries and is more lightweight. There are three manufacturers of thermal ablation devices, and they are already available in countries across all continents and income levels.

HPV POC test–based screening complemented with thermal ablation has the potential of a "one stop shop" for those women and individuals with a cervix that are eligible, providing an opportunity for cervical cancer screening in refugee and displaced populations, as it is a flexible setup that can be used in a myriad of circumstances and does not require highly specialized health personnel. It may also prove to be more easily integrable into other health services competing for limited resources and time of both health providers and women and individuals with a cervix.

It is important to note that implementation research is indispensable to guarantee the most effective and quality-assured services in different contexts.

3.7 Conclusion

Cervical cancer prevention (vaccination, screening, and treatment) is not generally included in healthcare for refugee and other forcibly displaced girls and women and individuals with a cervix, even though they seem to be at greater risk than the general population. In contexts where these services are available, there are multiple and overlapping barriers to accessing these services, but with the right messaging, and delivered in an inclusive, culturally safe and context-appropriate manner, there may be great potential to increase both vaccination and screening coverage in this underserved population. There are opportunities such as the one-dose vaccination schedule, the transition from conventional cytology or VIA to HPV-based screening, and the availability of transportable treatment devices to overcome barriers in different settings, but those will need increased efforts from policy makers, funders, developers, and manufacturers to be truly promising to ensure universal and equitable access to vaccines and CCS programs for all, irrespective of citizenship or migrant status.

References

Aantjes CJ, Govender K (2024) Are we getting any closer to including men and boys in sexual and reproductive health? A multi-country policy analysis on guidance to action in east and southern Africa. Int J Sex Health 36:464–483

Abdullahi A, Copping J, Kessel A, Luck M, Bonell C (2009) Cervical screening: perceptions and barriers to uptake among Somali women in Camden. Public Health 123:680–685

Allen EM, Lee HY, Pratt R, Vang H, Desai JR, Dube A et al (2019) Facilitators and barriers of cervical cancer screening and human papilloma virus vaccination among Somali refugee women in the United States: a qualitative analysis. J Transcult Nurs 30:55–63

Altaş ZM, Sezerol MA (2025) Migrant women's perception toward cervical and breast cancer screening in Türkiye: a qualitative analysis. BMC Public Health 25:190

Azerkan F, Widmark C, Sparén P, Weiderpass E, Tillgren P, Faxelid E (2015) When life got in the way: how Danish and Norwegian immigrant women in Sweden reason about cervical screening and why they postpone attendance. PLoS One 10:e0107624

Babatunde-Sowole OO, Power T, Davidson PM, DiGiacomo M, Jackson D (2020) Health screening and preventative health care in refugee women: a qualitative analysis. Contemp Nurse 56:62–79

Barrera-Castillo M, Fernández-Peña R, Del Valle-Gómez MDO, Fernández-Feito A, Lana A. Social integration and gynecologic cancer screening of immigrant women in Spain(2020) Gac Sanit 34:468–473

Bassett M, Writer S, Today M (2025) One dose of HPV vaccine noninferior to two, data show [web site]. https://www.medpagetoday.com/meetingcoverage/aacr/115340. Accessed 9 June 2025

Bray F, Laversanne M, Sung H, Ferlay J, Siegel RL, Soerjomataram I et al (2024) Global cancer statistics 2022: GLOBOCAN estimates of incidence and mortality worldwide for 36 cancers in 185 countries. CA Cancer J Clin 74:229–263

Cancer Today [web site]. (https://gco.iarc.who.int/today/. Accessed 4 Dec 2024

Casolino R, Sullivan R, Jobanputra K, Abdel-Wahab M, Grbic M, Hammad N et al (2025) Integrating cancer into crisis: a global vision for action from WHO and partners. Lancet Oncol 26:e55–e66

Cata-Preta BO, Santos TM, Wendt A, Arroyave L, Mengistu T, Hogan DR et al (2024) Inequalities in ownership and availability of home-based vaccination

records in 82 low- and middle-income countries. BMJ Glob Health 9:e016054
Cervical cancer [web site]. https://www.who.int/news-room/fact-sheets/detail/cervical-cancer. Accessed 8 Apr 2025
Costa T, Bateson D, Woo YL (2024) Enhancing equity in cervical screening—initiatives to increase screening participation. Curr Opin Obstet Gynecol 36:345
Davidson N, Hammarberg K, Romero L, Fisher J (2022) Access to preventive sexual and reproductive health care for women from refugee-like backgrounds: a systematic review. BMC Public Health 22:403
Ensuring the integration of refugees and migrants in immunization policies, planning and service delivery globally [web site]. https://www.who.int/publications/i/item/9789240051843. Accessed 7 June 2025
Garland SM, Bhatla N, Woo YL, Stanley M, Kaufmann A, Brotherton J et al (2024) IPVS STATEMENT on HPV vaccination: no longer supply constraints: towards achieving WHO vaccine targets. Vaccine 42:126400
Ghebrendrias S, Pfeil S, Crouthamel B, Chalmiers M, Kully G, Mody S (2021) An examination of misconceptions and their impact on cervical cancer prevention practices among sub-Saharan African and middle eastern refugees. Health Equity 5:382–389
Ghebreyesus TA, Mired D, Sullivan R, Mueller A, Charalambous A, Kacharian A et al (2024) A manifesto on improving cancer care in conflict-impacted populations. Lancet 404:427
Global strategy to accelerate the elimination of cervical cancer as a public health problem [web site]. https://www.who.int/publications/i/item/9789240014107. Accessed 21 Jan 2025
Guida F, Kidman R, Ferlay J, Schüz J, Soerjomataram I, Kithaka B et al (2022) Global and regional estimates of orphans attributed to maternal cancer mortality in 2020. Nat Med 28:2563–2572
Hadgkiss EJ, Renzaho AMN (2014) The physical health status, service utilisation and barriers to accessing care for asylum seekers residing in the community: a systematic review of the literature. Aust Health Rev Publ Aust Hosp Assoc 38:142–159
Hamdiui N, Marchena E, Stein ML, van Steenbergen JE, Crutzen R, van Keulen HM et al (2022) Decision-making, barriers, and facilitators regarding cervical cancer screening participation among Turkish and Moroccan women in The Netherlands: a focus group study. Ethn Health 27:1147–1165
Haworth RJ, Margalit R, Ross C, Nepal T, Soliman AS (2014) Knowledge, attitudes, and practices for cervical cancer screening among the Bhutanese refugee Community in Omaha. Nebraska J Commun Health 39:872–878
Hossain MA, Khanam SJ, Khan MN, Oldroyd J, Islam RM (2025) Barriers to cervical cancer screening among refugee women: a systematic review. PLOS Glob Public Health 5:e0004225
HPV Dashboard [web site]. https://www.who.int/teams/immunization-vaccines-and-biologicals/diseases/human-papillomavirus-vaccines-(HPV)/hpv-clearing-house/hpv-dashboard. Accessed 16 Apr 2025
https://www.unhcr.org/external/component/header [web site]. https://www.unhcr.org/external/component/header. Accessed 24 Apr 2025
Human papillomavirus vaccines: WHO position paper, December 2022 [web site]. https://www.who.int/publications/i/item/who-wer9750-645-672. Accessed 28 Nov 2024
Husain NE, Burhan A, Ahmed IAI, Mohammed SI, Hammad N (2022) Women's cancers in Sudan with a focus on cervical cancer: turmoil, geopolitics and opportunities. Ecancermedicalscience 16:1433
Kim K, Kim S, Chung Y (2017) A qualitative study exploring factors associated with Pap test use among North Korean refugees. Health Care Women Int 38:1115–1129
Knights F, Carter J, Deal A, Crawshaw A, Bouaddi O, Sanchez-Clemente N et al (2024) Strengthening life-course immunisation in migrant populations: access, equity, and inclusion. Lancet Reg Health – Eur 41:100806
Kue J, Hanegan H, Tan A (2017) Perceptions of cervical cancer screening, screening behavior, and post-migration living difficulties among Bhutanese–Nepali refugee women in the United States. J Community Health 42:1079–1089
Lilleston P, Winograd L, Ahmed S, Salamé D, Al Alam D, Stoebenau K et al (2018) Evaluation of a mobile approach to gender-based violence service delivery among Syrian refugees in Lebanon. Health Policy Plan 33:767–776
Lor B, Ornelas IJ, Magarati M, Do HH, Zhang Y, Jackson JC et al (2018) We should know ourselves: Burmese and Bhutanese refugee women's perspectives on cervical cancer screening. J Health Care Poor Underserved 29:881–897
Marques P, Nunes M, Antunes M d L, Heleno B, Dias S (2020) Factors associated with cervical cancer screening participation among migrant women in Europe: a scoping review. Int J Equity Health 19:160
McLeroy KR, Bibeau D, Steckler A, Glanz K (1988) An ecological perspective on health promotion programs. Health Educ Q 15:351–377
Milenkov AR, Felini M, Baker E, Acharya R, Diese EL, Onsa S et al (2020) Uptake of cancer screenings among a multiethnic refugee population in North Texas, 2014-2018. PLoS One 15:e0230675
Ngwibete A, Ogunbode O, Oluwasola T, Omigbodun A (2024) Provision of sexual and reproductive health services to internally displaced women and refugees in Africa: a systematic review. Malawi Med J 36:238–249
O'Donnell CA, Burns N, Mair FS, Dowrick C, Clissmann C, van den Muijsenbergh M et al (2016) Reducing the health care burden for marginalised migrants: the potential role for primary care in Europe. Health Policy 120:495–508
Organization WH (2016) Guide to introducing HPV vaccine into national immunization programmes.

World Health Organization. https://iris.who.int/handle/10665/253123. Accessed 7 July 2025

Ou L, Chen AC-C, Amresh A (2023) The effectiveness of mHealth interventions targeting parents and youth in human papillomavirus vaccination: systematic review. JMIR Pediatr Parent 6:e47334

Pannetier J, Ravalihasy A, Lydié N, Lert F, du Loû AD (2018) Protecting female migrants from forced sex and HIV infection. Lancet Public Health 3:e112

Parajuli J, Horey, Dell, Avgoulas M-I (2020) Perceived barriers to cervical cancer screening among refugee women after resettlement: a qualitative study. Contemp Nurse 56:363–375

Poljak M, Oštrbenk Valenčak A, Cuschieri K, Bohinc KB, Arbyn M (2024) 2023 global inventory of commercial molecular tests for human papillomaviruses (HPV). J Clin Virol 172:105671

Report on the health of refugees and migrants in the WHO European Region: no public health without refugee and migrant health (2018) [web site]. https://www.who.int/publications/i/item/report-on-the-health-of-refugees-and-migrants-in-the-who-european-region-no-public-health-without-refugee-and-migrant-health. Accessed 31 May 2025

Schliemann D, Tan MM, Hoe WMK, Mohan D, Taib NA, Donnelly M et al (2022) mHealth interventions to improve cancer screening and early detection: scoping review of reviews. J Med Internet Res 24:e36316

Snapshot. https://www.gavi.org/types-support/vaccine-support/human-papillomavirus. Accessed 24 Apr 2025

Strengthening Health Initiatives: WHO Representative a.i. to Bangladesh's Impactful Visit to Cox's Bazar [web site]. https://www.who.int/bangladesh/news/detail/10-03-2025-strengthening-health-initiatives-who-representative-ai-to-bangladesh-impactful-visit-to-cox-s-bazar. Accessed 8 July 2025

Tazinya RMA, El-Mowafi IM, Hajjar JM, Yaya S (2023) Sexual and reproductive health and rights in humanitarian settings: a matter of life and death. Reprod Health 20:42

Troisi G, Gafer N, Alsawahli H, Elmusharaf K, Byström M, Azar J et al (2025) Harnessing primary healthcare to reduce the burden of cervical cancer in the eastern Mediterranean region. BMJ Glob Health 10:e017622

Turkey: MoH/SIHHAT – surveys for health care needs analysis of Syrian population under temporary protection [web site]. https://data.unhcr.org/en/documents/details/88643. Accessed 7 Feb 2025

UNHCR, the UN Refugee Agency [web site]. https://www.unhcr.org/. Accessed 15 Apr 2025

van Loenen T, van den Muijsenbergh M, Hofmeester M, Dowrick C, van Ginneken N, Mechili EA et al (2018) Primary care for refugees and newly arrived migrants in Europe: a qualitative study on health needs, barriers and wishes. Eur J Pub Health 28:82–87

Walker PF, Settgast AM, DeSilva MB (2022) Cancer screening in refugees and immigrants: a global perspective. Am J Trop Med Hyg 106:1593–1600

Whitworth HS, Mounier-Jack S, Choi EM, Gallagher KE, Howard N, Kelly H et al (2024) Efficacy and immunogenicity of a single dose of human papillomavirus vaccine compared to multidose vaccination regimens or no vaccination: an updated systematic review of evidence from clinical trials. Vaccine X 19:100486

WHO HPV Vaccine Global Market Study, April 2022 [web site]. https://www.who.int/publications/m/item/who-hpv-vaccine-global-market-study-april-2022. Accessed 17 Apr 2025

WHO Immunization Data portal – Global [web site]. https://immunizationdata.who.int. Accessed 7 July 2025

Wong HY, Wong EL-Y (2024) Invitation strategy of vaginal HPV self-sampling to improve participation in cervical cancer screening: a systematic review and meta-analysis of randomized trials. BMC Public Health 24:2461

World Health Organization (2014) Comprehensive cervical cancer control: a guide to essential practice, 2nd edn. World Health Organization, Geneva. https://iris.who.int/handle/10665/144785. Accessed 30 Apr 2025

World Health Organization (2019) WHO guidelines for the use of thermal ablation for cervical pre-cancer lesions. World Health Organization, Geneva. https://iris.who.int/handle/10665/329299. Accessed 28 Nov 2024

World Health Organization (2021a) Special Programme of research, development, and research training in human reproduction (World Health Organization). WHO guideline for screening and treatment of cervical pre-cancer lesions for cervical cancer prevention, 2nd edn. World Health Organization, Geneva

World Health Organization (2021b) WHO guideline for screening and treatment of cervical pre-cancer lesions for cervical cancer prevention: use of MRNA tests for Human Papillomavirus (HPV), 2nd edn. World Health Organization, Geneva

World Health Organization (2024) Target product profiles for human papillomavirus screening tests to detect cervical pre-cancer and cancer. World health Organization. https://iris.who.int/handle/10665/379099. Accessed 4 Dec 2024

World report on the health of refugees and migrants [web site]. https://www.who.int/publications/i/item/9789240054462. Accessed 12 Dec 2024

Zhang Y, Ornelas IJ, Do HH, Magarati M, Jackson JC, Taylor VM (2017) Provider perspectives on promoting cervical cancer screening among refugee women. J Community Health 42:583–590

Borders, Barriers, and Violence: Healthcare Challenges in (Migrant) Sex Work

4

Isotta Rossoni and Jonathan Camilleri

Contents

Abstract

Research on sex work in Malta is, to date, limited. In this chapter, the authors draw on two complementary qualitative research studies involving 46 participants with lived experiences of sex work to explore the barriers sex workers face in accessing healthcare and ancillary services in Malta. Using Levesque et al.'s (Int J Equity Health 12, 1: 18, 2013) "access to healthcare" framework, findings are presented paying particular attention to the testimonies of migrant sex workers and help-seeking following violence.

I. Rossoni (✉)
Van Vollenhoven Institute -Leiden Law School, Leiden University, Leiden, The Netherlands

J. Camilleri
Department of Security and Crime Science, University College London, London, UK
e-mail: j.camilleri.17@ucl.ac.uk

V. Padovese, I. Rossoni (eds.), *Intersections of Sexual Health, Migration and Sexualised Violence*, Sustainable Development Goals Series, https://doi.org/10.1007/978-3-032-20707-4_4

The results discussed in this chapter highlight that many migrant sex workers face significant challenges in accessing sexual health services in Malta, including following experiences of violence. Hurdles such as strict residency and taxation requirements for HIV treatment, as well as the reliance on private healthcare due to delays in public health services, remain particularly problematic. Moreover, sex-work, gender and race-related biases among practitioners have a bearing on access to dignified care for all sex workers, especially in cases of sexual and other violence experienced during sex work. When gender intersects with precarious migrant status, violence may often remain hidden, as fear of repercussions deters migrant sex workers from seeking help or speaking out.

The authors strongly emphasise the need to move beyond restrictive policy arrangements on sex work that negatively impact sex workers' health. They further underscore the importance of targeted training for professionals on working with (migrant) sex workers, and call for research that can further investigate the role of peer education in access to health, aiming to build a stronger evidence base for targeted interventions.

Keywords

Sex work · Migration · Access to health · Agency · Malta · Decriminalisation · Policy-making

4.1 Introduction

Sex workers are a heterogeneous group of people (Weitzer 2012), who provide their "own sexual labour" in exchange for money, goods or other resources (Smith and Mac 2018). This exchange "occurs across a constantly shifting spectrum of choice, circumstance, and coercion" (Albright and D'Adamo 2017). How sex work should or should not be framed remains contentious in academia, policy and practice, and critics challenge the perspective that sex work can be work, arguing that sex work cannot be equated with other forms of labour due to its potential for exploitation (Raymond 2013; Farley 1994). Others have argued that sex work is often no more harmful than many commonly accepted occupations. If sex work "is consensual, worker-controlled, non-abusive, and no more exploitative than the average job would be" (Moen 2014), it can be a valid occupational choice though criminalisation and repression may undermine these conditions (Vanwesenbeeck 2017). These scholars have demonstrated that attempts at abolishing or criminalising aspects of sex work may also "fundamentally violate people's right to professional, sexual, and bodily agency and self-determination" (Vanwesenbeeck 2017).

Due to the widespread normative debates which surround sex work—and unlike many other forms of labour—sex work remains "widely stigmatised" (Nussbaum 1998), resulting in significant social, legal and economic challenges for those who engage in it, including barriers to accessing legal, medical or social services. Intersecting vulnerabilities may exacerbate already significant difficulties to access needed services. For migrant sex workers, for example, racism and xenophobia (McBride and Janushev 2021) may play an important role in the way they are or expect to be treated, while disparate border regimes (Vuolajärvi 2019) may expose them to surveillance, detention and even deportation under the language of anti-trafficking activities. This framing often leads to undermining sex workers' autonomy and can also contribute to systemic violence against this already vulnerabilised group. Policies rooted in abolitionist ideologies, for example, often propose to criminalise clients or third parties (Raymond 2003), which may displace sex work further outside of visible spaces. In doing so, sex workers may be increasingly exposed to unsafe conditions and take increased risks (Krüsi et al. 2014), while limiting their ability to report abuse or access legal protections without fear of prosecution or stigma. Additionally, the conflation of sex work with trafficking perpetuates stereotypes that deny agency to sex workers (Thomas 2021) and may often result in interventions that prioritise "rescue" rather than addressing the systemic barriers they face using agent-centric approaches.

Healthcare is an area where these intersecting challenges are very acute. Sex workers may face barriers accessing health services, including fear of exposure, fear of criminal repercussions or victim-blaming (Goldenberg et al. 2021). Language barriers, precarious legal statuses and limited understanding of available services and their rights can also magnify existing barriers (Faissner et al. 2024). These systemic barriers may often lead to unmet health needs, increased vulnerability to violence, and overall, poorer health outcomes. Violence against sex workers has been widely documented, be it from clients, procurers, law enforcement or broader society or institutions (Deering et al. 2014). Stigma, dehumanising behaviour or even outright denial of care experienced when attempting to access healthcare services can itself be a form of violence and further pushes to the margins an already marginalised group (Benoit et al. 2018).

In this chapter, we draw on two complementary studies conducted by the authors, both involving participants with lived experiences of sex work (see Camilleri and Rossoni 2026). We present our analysis of some key findings on the barriers Maltese and migrant sex workers face in accessing healthcare and ancillary services in Malta. We explore these barriers with a particular focus on the additional challenges faced by migrant sex workers and their specific needs. These studies provide a rich foundation for the discussion, and the different methods used will be explained in greater detail in the methods section of this chapter. To set the stage, we first provide an overview of the context surrounding sex work in Malta, with a focus on its legal and policy framework. We then discuss violence in (migrant) sex work, before providing an explanation of the methodologies employed in both studies and the theoretical framework utilised in this chapter. This is followed by an analysis of barriers to healthcare access, particularly in cases of violence, using Levesque et al.'s "access to healthcare" framework to explore the interplay of structural constraints and individual agency, with a focus on migrant sex workers (Levesque et al. 2013). Through a synthesis of insights from individual analytical perspectives, we offer commentary on these findings and conclude with actionable recommendations for policy and practice.

4.2 Sex Work in Malta: Law and Policy

Sex work in Malta escapes a clear-cut legal definition. Although sex work per se is not illegal, Maltese law criminalises a range of acts which are tightly related to the sale of sexual services. The Civil Code provides for the termination of rental agreements when the premises are being used for "prostitution or other immoral purposes" (Government of Malta 2024a). Moreover, although not formulated exactly as such by law, sharing a dwelling where sexual services are being sold is often considered by the courts as running a brothel and punished accordingly (Monique Agius 2022, 2023). Additionally, the law allows to disinherit any descendants who are found to engage in prostitution (Government of Malta n.d.). Forced prostitution, trafficking, living off the profits of the prostitution of a minor and solicitation/loitering are prohibited under the Criminal Code (Government of Malta 2024b). Trafficking is also regulated by the White Slave Ordinance (Government of Malta 2007).

In recent years, sex work regulations in Malta have come under increased scrutiny, raising the prospect of legal reform. In 2019, the Government of Malta announced a public consultation for the revision of sex work and trafficking legislation and policy inviting submissions from experts, academics, civil society organisations and other interested parties (Government of Malta 2019). The proposed reform had the twin aspiration of developing a comprehensive National Strategy Against Human Trafficking whilst concurrently decriminalising the sex industry. It is worth noting that the consultation document used the terms "legalisation" and "decriminalisation" of sex work interchangeably, making the government's exact intentions unclear. As these terms reflect distinct legal frameworks for sex work

(International Women's Rights Action Watch Asia Pacific 2017), it was not immediately evident towards which approach the government was leaning. Following the Covid-19 pandemic taking centre-stage and the Parliamentary Secretary tasked with leading the process stepping down, discussions surrounding the reform fell off the political agenda as quickly as they had emerged. To date, sex work legislation in Malta remains unaltered and nebulous, failing to clearly articulate the rights of sex workers.

4.3 Violence in the Context of (Migrant) Sex Work

While there is still limited research exploring sex work in Malta, and even less about violence within the migrant sex working community in Malta (Scicluna and Clark 2019; Rossoni et al. 2022; Rossoni and Van der Woude 2025; Rossoni 2026a), internationally, violence in the context of sex work has been well documented both by academic research and sex worker-led initiatives (SWERV: Sex Workers Evaluate Reporting Violence—National Ugly Mugs 2025; ESWA Applauds the Position of the UN Working Group on Discrimination against Women and Girls 2025; Kloek et al. 2024; Ślęzak 2018). Existing data indicates that framing violence against sex workers as being an "occupational hazard" oversimplifies the issue, as it is actually driven by a complex interplay of intersecting factors. Experiences of violence are fuelled by a diverse range of factors, including legal policies and the regulation of sex work, workplace conditions, gender inequalities, power dynamics, societal stigmatisation of sex work, migration patterns, the sexual coercion of women and girls, as well as interpersonal, individual, and psychosocial influences (Deering et al. 2014).

Notwithstanding the coexistence of a multitude of factors associated or correlated with violence, as underlined by numerous studies, a leading role can be attributed to legal and policy aspects (Oliveira et al. 2023; Grenfell et al. 2023; Calderaro and Giametta 2019). Regarding the legal and policy dimension, Deering et al. (2014) in their systematic review of international literature on violence and sex work, highlighted the harmful consequences of enforcing partial or total criminalisation. In contexts where clients are criminalised, those willing to risk legal penalties for purchasing sexual services are often the most ruthless individuals—those with "less to lose" and, consequently, the most likely to engage in abusive behaviour (Smith and Mac 2018). Moreover, in some countries, repressive policing not only leads to higher rates of client-perpetrated violence but also contributes to increased incidents of police violence. From a labour-dimension, the authors emphasised that street-based sex work is particularly hazardous compared to other forms of sex work (Lynzi 2019; Penfold et al. 2004; Rosie et al. 2020). Additionally, economic pressures were identified as exacerbating sex workers' vulnerability to abuse, both from clients and, in some cases, from intimate partners (Jansson et al. 2023).

Gender equality and social stigma were discussed as both protective and risk factors, with the latter being prominent in societies characterised by significant inequalities and conservative attitudes towards sex work. Similarly, interpersonal, individual and psychosocial factors were recognised as playing dual roles, acting as both safeguards against violence and contributors to it. Consistent with numerous other studies, migration—whether voluntary or coerced—was found to heighten exposure to violence (Rocha-Jiménez et al. 2016; Modupe-Oluwa and Heumann 2014; McBride et al. 2020; Sampethai 2022). Beyond cases where sex workers migrate under the promise of decent working conditions only to face exploitation upon arrival (Hughes 2000; Liu 2012), the research underscored the profound power imbalances stemming from the lack of legal migration status. Irregular status can often be exploited by clients, enabling them to perpetrate abuse without fear of accountability (McBride et al. 2020). A more recent UK-based qualitative study corroborated several of these findings, particularly regarding the detrimental impact of harmful policies and practices (Grenfell et al. 2023). Through in-depth interviews with nearly 50 sex workers in London, the study revealed that enforcement practices by police, immigration authorities and even support services collaborating with the government adversely affected sex workers' working conditions, intensifying their precarity and exposure to violence. The few support services that were genuinely valued by sex workers were significantly underfunded. Conversely, most public services for sex workers operated under "safe communities" principles, which further marginalised sex workers and increased their potential exposure to violence.

Particularly relevant to this chapter are studies examining the linkages between policies, violence and health. A 2018 systematic review and meta-analysis of quantitative and qualitative research in this areas highlighted that repressive policing practices targeting sex workers are linked to higher rates of sexual and physical violence perpetrated by clients or other partners (Platt et al. 2018). Furthermore, sex workers subjected to such policing face increased risks of contracting HIV and other sexually transmitted infections (STIs), largely due to the higher prevalence of condomless sex in contexts where sex work is partially or fully criminalised. The study also underscored the significant impact of criminalisation on access to healthcare and, more broadly, fundamental rights. These findings align with research from the EU context (Oliveira et al. 2023), which makes a compelling case that the criminalisation of sex work infringes on sex workers' right to health, undermining prevention, testing and treatment for STIs and HIV, as well as their overall mental health. Migrant sex workers may often face heightened challenges in these environments. Beyond the stigma associated with sex work (Lazarus et al. 2012), they encounter additional barriers linked to migration, such as unfamiliarity with available services, language and cultural barriers, and restricted access to treatment due to their migration status (Rita et al. 2022). These compounded vulnerabilities further exacerbate their hardship and limit their ability to seek essential support.

4.4 Methods

Empirical research on sex work and its potential intersections with exploitation and human trafficking poses significant logistical and ethical challenges, largely because its subjects are members of so-called "hidden populations" (Shaver 2005; Zhang et al. 2014). Such groups cannot be "readily distinguished or enumerated based on existing knowledge and/or sampling capabilities" (Wiebel 1998), while "public acknowledgement of membership in the population is potentially threatening" (Heckathorn 1997a). Moreover, many research subjects in these fields can also be members of multiple or intersecting hidden groups, such as "injecting drug users, men who have sex with men, and the homeless", all of whom share privacy concerns based on the stigma they are often subject to (Heckathorn 1997b). In tight-knit communities, such as in the Maltese setting, experiences and effects of stigma may be more acute (Kada 2019; Crumb et al. 2019).

4.4.1 Trust and Sensitivity

Beyond the difficulties of locating and accessing participants, researchers must carefully balance addressing participants' "tacit mistrust of outsiders" while avoiding the risk of participants feeling intimidated or "interrogated on their possible criminal activity"—especially for researchers in criminology or crime science (Elgabry and Camilleri 2021). Even then, broaching experiences of exploitation or victimization and other delicate subjects can be an additional hurdle in and of itself (Elmir et al. 2011). To address the lack of evidence on sex work in Malta and demonstrate that these challenges can be overcome in the local context, the authors of this chapter conducted separate but complementary studies, employing methodologies that prioritised participant safety and inclusivity to enhance understanding of this complex issue.

4.4.2 Two Studies, One Goal: Understanding Sex Work in Malta

The first author conducted a study in collaboration with Malta's only public sexual health clinic, which offers free STI and HIV testing to Maltese citizens, EU nationals and non-EU residents (see Rossoni 2026b). This collaboration facilitated access to migrant sex workers from diverse regions, including Europe, South America, and Asia. The researcher was present at the clinic during working hours to recruit participants and also conducted outreach activities at refugee and asylum seeker centres to facilitate access to both testing services and research participation. The research sample ($n = 29$) consisted of 25 migrant sex workers—engaging in sex work either casually or as full-time occupation—aged 18 and older, encompassing diverse genders, sexual orientations, nationalities, and migration statuses, and 4 Maltese participants including a pimp and 3 sex workers. One participant was interviewed twice, before and after entering a social protection programme for survivors of trafficking. Snowball sampling was employed to expand the participant pool. Fieldwork was conducted during intensive research stints over approximately 1 year (2022–2023), and data collection employed a combination of semi-structured interviews and photo elicitation. Participants received free sexual health kits as a token of appreciation, ensuring ethical acknowledgment of their contributions without compromising integrity.

The second author's study involved a series of interviews with sex workers who had lived or worked in Malta and were fluent in either Maltese or English. This research was part of a broader, dual-track project that also included interviews with non-sex-working stakeholders (see Camilleri 2025). Recruitment took place over a 7-month period, from 2022 to early 2023, employing a mix of online and offline strategies such as social media advertisements and printed flyers distributed at strategic locations across Malta. Efforts were made at the recruitment stage to ensure inclusivity, engaging participants from diverse backgrounds, including varying genders, sexual orientations and nationalities. Snowball sampling was also utilised to expand the participant pool (Faugier and Sargeant 1997). Data collection centred on event-based narratives, exploring how participants ($n = 17$) navigated their work over time through in-depth, semi-structured interviews (Guest et al. 2013; King et al. 2019). This method combined semi-structured interviews with event-based approaches, encouraging participants to share their experiences and actions naturally through storytelling. Participants were compensated to acknowledge their time, contributions and opportunity costs (Ripley 2006; Head 2009; Camilleri et al. 2025). To ensure comfort and mitigate bias, interviews with cis- and trans-female participants included a trusted female psychotherapist, fostering a safe and supportive environment.

In both studies, interviews were transcribed in an edited verbatim format omitting or anonymising personally identifiable information (Heaton 2022). All recordings and transcripts were securely stored in encrypted folders. Participants in both studies were fully informed about confidentiality measures and their voluntary participation rights through clear oral explanations and detailed information sheets. Specific precautions were tailored to each study: the first author ensured participation was entirely unrelated to access to health services, removing any pressure to participate, while the second author used an opt-out approach to compensation, automatically compensating participants unless they declined, regardless of their contribution.

4.4.3 Theoretical Framework

The data analysis was guided by Levesque et al.'s "access to healthcare" framework, which adopts a strengths-based approach to individual agency while acknowledging the structural and societal constraints that limit access. The authors privileged this model over others for its ability to highlight the wealth of resources and skills sex workers draw upon to navigate challenges in accessing health and rights, rather than focusing solely on the barriers migrant sex workers face.

The "access to healthcare" framework recognises that there are five dimensions of accessibility of services, which include approachability (transparency, outreach, information, screening), acceptability (professional values, norms, culture and gender), availability and accommodation (geographic location, hours of opening, accommodation, appointment mechanisms), affordability (direct and indirect costs, opportunity costs) and appropriateness (technical and interpersonal quality, adequacy, coordination and continuity) (Levesque et al. 2013). Each dimension is paired with corresponding abilities—skills that enable individuals to navigate these dimensions and achieve access (Levesque et al. 2013). This chapter uses the framework to explore factors influencing sex workers' access to (sexual) healthcare, particularly following experiences of violence. The analysis primarily focuses on migrant sex workers, with occasional comparisons to Maltese sex workers to highlight the unique impact of migratory journeys on access.

4.4.4 Limitations

This chapter is based on two separate research projects, each with its own limitations that must be taken into account when interpreting the findings.

Despite the authors' best efforts to engage a diverse range of participants, sex workers—being a hidden and often stigmatised population—may be hesitant to take part in such research (Shaver 2005). As a result, the reliance on snowball sampling, direct outreach, and advertising may have introduced selection bias, favouring individuals more willing to share their experiences (Atkinson and Flint 2011). Neither project aimed to produce statistically generalisable findings but instead focused on generating depth of understanding. Consequently, the findings should not be taken to represent all sex workers in Malta, nor do they fully capture the varied and nuanced experiences of different subgroups within the community, both known and unknown. Specifically, in relation to migrant sex workers, localised outreach may have inadvertently skewed the sample towards individuals already connected to support services, although snowball sampling partially mitigated this issue (Padovese et al. 2021; Rossoni et al. 2023; Oriol et al. 2023). Additionally, language and cultural differences may have influenced data collection and the responses of participants, despite the authors' concerted efforts to minimise these barriers (Li 2011).

While both studies included healthcare within a broader investigation of themes such as decision-making, vulnerability and economic factors, they were not specifically designed to focus solely on healthcare access. The findings, therefore, provide a snapshot of participants' concerns rather than a holistic analysis but offer a valuable foundation for future research to address these gaps. Despite this, the chapter highlights critical barriers faced by sex workers in Malta, particularly migrants, and underscores the need for policy and service reforms to improve their rights, healthcare access, and overall well-being.

4.4.5 Funding Statement

The research discussed in this chapter, specifically the second author's contributions, was partially funded by the Tertiary Education Scholarships Scheme (Malta). All aspects of the research were conducted independently, without editorial input or oversight from the funding body. The funding covered academic fees and travel expenses, with all other costs borne by the author.

4.5 From Evidence to Insight

4.5.1 Approachability

Approachability comprises both the propensity of health institutions to make themselves known via the provision of accurate and reliable information about available services and outreach, and the ability of migrant populations to perceive a need for care. The latter is generally influenced by health literacy and beliefs around health, well-being and sickness (Levesque et al. 2013).

Research on access to sexual health in Europe and Malta testifies to migrants presenting late to services and generally seeking care only when symptoms present themselves, rather than for preventive purposes (Padovese et al. 2021). Most participants in this study had sufficient knowledge of existing sexual health services on the island, though may not necessarily have made use of them. This should come as no surprise, as a large percentage of them were individuals who had lived in Malta for a while and had already accessed the island's only public sexual health clinic, often as a result of an ongoing sexual health issue requiring treatment. Regardless of this, participants' responses suggested that a key factor shaping approachability is sex workers' own sense of self-care, which in turn impacted their perceived *need* for care. While self-care was broadly acknowledged as a prerequisite for staying safe while selling sexual services (Turcotte and Lanctôt 2021), participants qualified it in slightly different ways based on their views, personal history and experiences.

For AR, a sex worker who relocated to Malta a few years ago from a neighbouring European country, safety meant prioritising his bodily integrity and minimising health risks. He emphasised the importance of limiting certain activities he deemed "riskier", such as specific sexual acts, to trusted individuals and avoiding situations involving blood or sex under the influence of drugs.[1]

> What is absurd in sex? Honestly, very little (…) There are many games (…), the kind of things that you do with people you know because you need a certain level of security and to look after your health. Avoid having your hands tied because you never know how someone may react and they might fly off the handle. Chemsex can lead to mood swings… I have three hard no's: cleanliness, blood and extreme pain. (AR)

AR's account highlights the influence of beliefs about sex—what is deemed acceptable, with whom and under what circumstances—on sex workers' understanding of self-care. His testimony demonstrates that health-related and other "risks" are often navigated based on personal perceptions of safety or, conversely, feelings of insecurity (Lawan et al. 2012). For LO, a Latin-American HIV-positive patient, "caring" about health carried a stronger normative dimension, approaching a moral imperative. LO was concerned about his health and perceived it as influencing various aspects of his life, including his migration decisions.

> I have [emphasis in original] to care about it [my health], which is why during COVID I had to stay here… (LO)

Building further on LO's notion of self-care as a moral duty, JA, a Maltese sex worker, emphasised that self-care also involves a responsibility towards others. In her view, this responsibility is not limited to sex workers but applies to anyone who engages in sexual activity without being "*care*-ful" [emphasis added].

> Even though I've been doing this job for 13 years, I've always done my health screening. I've never had an infection. I mean, there are those who say prostitutes spread disease: not at all if you careful, because I haven't had anything in twelve years. No chlamydia or gonorrhoea, nothing. So, it depends on the person. If it isn't a prostitute, it could be a lowly person, like you don't do the job [but] you hook up, have sex and do it every day and don't use [contraception]. You don't have to be a prostitute or whatever. (JA)

These testimonies suggest that sexual health services in Malta may be "approachable," in that they are generally recognised by both locals and migrants. However, this approachability, and the perceived need for care, seems to be shaped by sex workers' personal interpretations of self-care, which are influenced by their beliefs about sex and their sense of duty of care towards themselves and others.

[1] Pseudonyms are used throughout.

4.5.2 Acceptability

Acceptability encompasses cultural and social factors, such as the gender, ethnicity or other relevant identity markers of providers, alongside the beliefs and norms governing the health system. It hinges on the service's capacity to address the complex and diverse needs of all patients, including minorities and marginalised groups, in a manner sensitive to their specific needs and realities. The ability to seek healthcare, meanwhile, relies on personal autonomy, the capacity to make decisions about accessing care and awareness of health and individual rights (Levesque et al. 2013). As Levesque et al. concede, it can be difficult for services to fully grasp and accommodate the different and often intersectional needs of a diverse patient population. Even within the migrant cohort of the combined data-set, service acceptability was judged differently based on personal experience, perceptions of racism towards one's national/ethnic group or comparison with one's country of origin (Levesque et al. 2013).

MM, who relocated to Malta from another European country several years ago, regarded the healthcare system as generally "very good" compared to that of his home country. Similarly, JR, from South-East Asia, also commended the "health sections for being good compared to my country." However, he observed that his perception of the acceptability of healthcare and other institutions improved as he became more integrated into Maltese society, partly due to his steady relationship with a local. In contrast, LO from Latin America was highly critical of the functioning of the health system, highlighting the impact that preconceived norms around race have, in his view, on the provision of information to patients.

> I went to the hospital because I had some sexual health problems, because I suffer some reaction, my immunity is going down, last week. I was fucked, completely fucked. I texted them one day before for the nurse at hospital by email... because almost 1 year that I don't go there, because when I went there they told me I have to pay a lot... I discovered now that I don't have to pay. Racist, racism in Malta, they have a lot. They want to take money from every side! (LO)

Experiences of violence revealed a complex interplay between the "ability to seek care" and the capacity of healthcare services to provide dignified treatment to survivors, as highlighted in several interviews. The majority of participants, including most migrant participants too, reported incidents of physical or sexual violence by clients. However, in the vast majority of cases—almost unilaterally—health services were not sought, and even then not necessarily within close temporal proximity to the incident. Moreover, participants across the board tended not to report violence. For locals, this appeared to be the result of mistrust in the police, fear of stigmatisation or victim-blaming, and was treated as an "occupational hazard" (Struyf 2023). For migrants, these issues were exacerbated by fears that reporting would have repercussions on their right to remain in the country. This underscores a general tendency to "keep a low profile," particularly amongst marginalised groups and even more so among those with insecure migration status.

The testimony of BE, a local sex worker who sought care at A&E after experiencing violence at the hands of a client, which had a long-term impact on her health going forward, highlights the detrimental impact of gender-related and other stereotypes on access to healthcare services in Malta. Reflecting the experiences of female sex worker survivors documented in international research, she recounted how the attending medical professional downplayed the violence she had endured and failed to fulfil his duty of care, including by refusing to provide appropriate sexual health testing. She also concealed that she was engaging in sex work at the time of her assault, because she did not feel at ease disclosing this information.

> This was with a particular client (...) so what happened was that he took me back to his place, and kind of pinned me down, did what he did, wore no contraceptives and I was really worried, and basically I just took myself to the hospital. I don't know how I got myself out of his place, but, I did. I ran two whole blocks, then called a cab, got into the cab (...). I was on the table, and when the doctor came and asked me questions, he told me 'But you knew this person?', and I told him, 'I met him.'

> And he told me, 'but did you consent to have relations with this person?' And then I told him, 'Yes, but...' And when I said 'Yes', he kind of stopped me there and said, 'Listen, you barely have any bruising. You just have a couple of hairs pulled.' Like, bruising developed much later, for instance. He told me like, 'A broken lip is barely anything. I'm not going to check you. It's a waste of my time.' And basically I was kind of like told to fuck off. And basically I decided to go to the closest pharmacy I can, find one which is open, and go the morning after pill, and basically took that, cleaned myself up and continued on... (BE)

Participants' testimonies revealed that the acceptability of sexual health services can be undermined by various factors, including healthcare providers' gendered beliefs about sexual and other forms of violence, exacerbated by biases against sex work, and prejudices related to race and ethnicity.

Being a migrant was not always a barrier to accessing care: acceptability could be influenced by the length of the migrant's stay in the country, the degree of racism experienced by their perceived ethnic group and the extent to which migrants view healthcare in the home country as better or worse compared to the host country. However, an unstable migration status consistently acted as a barrier, preventing sex-working survivors of violence from reporting abuse and seeking care or support.

4.5.3 Availability and Accommodation

Availability and accommodation refer to the ease with which health services can be reached. "Reachability" is primarily influenced geography (i.e. where services are located, proximity to transport options, building accessibility) as well as practical considerations like opening hours. Conversely, the ability to access care is affected by factors such as the distance of one's accommodation from urban areas, ease of access to transportation, flexibility in work arrangements, and the presence of disabilities or other personal circumstances (Levesque et al. 2013).

A significant factor positively influencing the availability of sexual health services in Malta is the provision of confidential, anonymous and free access to public sexual health services at the genito-urinary clinic (GUC), irrespective of migration status.[2] Moreover, due to the island's relatively small size, geographical barriers were not identified as a significant issue. Nonetheless, participants highlighted other concerns that, in their view, impact service availability and accessibility. BW, a non-EU citizen, discussed the challenges of accessing general healthcare services, including sexual and reproductive health services not covered by the GUC, in the absence of a valid ID. More specifically, she expressed her doubts about the healthcare system's ability to accommodate her, even if she were to prove that she is, in fact, fulfilling her tax obligations.

> It's difficult. I mean thankfully, I haven't gotten sick or anything. If I go to the hospital, I can show that I pay tax and if they see that I pay NI or health security then I get the services. But it's always better if I have my ID card. Like I haven't tried without my ID Card but I'm pretty sure that ... I might need to go to the private hospital. (BW)

In a similar manner, YA, a migrant from a European country, acknowledged that they currently enjoy access to healthcare because they are paying tax, yet expressed concern over the possibility of losing this privilege, were they to become unemployed.

> When it comes to medical (...) the government pays me because I am paying a tax, you know the national insurance (...). That's the point, but I work for it. If I don't have a full time job then I don't have access to it. (YA)

Similarly, regarding HIV treatment, which in Malta is fully reliant on tax contributions and residency status,[3] AS—a migrant from Latin America—spoke of having to fend for himself when the system failed to accommodate his needs. He also highlighted the health risks associated with having to obtain treatment through alternative means.

> And I had to spend another 2 months without medication and that left me very worried (...) In the

[2] For further information see: https://sexualhealth.gov.mt/mt/node/753

[3] See: https://www.hivmalta.com/travelling-to-malta

> end the only solution I could find was to buy it. I have papers but to be able to access the treatment I have to show 3 payslips. This pill gave me headaches, and I've never had a headache in my life, it gave me pain in my eyes and it causes the white of the eye to turn orange… night sweats. (AS)[4]

Participants' accounts indicated that the primary factors affecting access to healthcare for migrant sex workers, particularly access to HIV treatment, are residency status and stringent taxation requirements. In a context where selling sex is technically legal but not recognised as official employment, the inability to secure regular employment significantly hinders access to healthcare for migrant sex workers.

4.5.4 Affordability

Affordability relates to services' accessibility from a financial perspective, and concurrently to individuals' ability to invest resources and time to access healthcare. Purchasing power is not immutable and may be affected by factors such as ease of access to employment, events leading to lifestyle changes, broader societal crises and even global phenomena (Levesque et al. 2013). Similar to acceptability, affordability was assessed by some participants in comparison to their home countries. Malta was particularly praised for providing free sexual health services.

> Compared and I can say about the [home country] because in [home country] the treatment for the venereal disease they are not included in the insurance and stuff. (MM)
> The only thing is that the health sections are very good, free and good compared to my country. (JR)

Nevertheless, attention was drawn to the cost of HIV treatment for individuals who do not have residency, are not paying taxes, and therefore cannot access the free HIV treatment available to taxpayers.

> The one [pill] I am telling you about costs more than 1000 euros, there is another pill that has many side effects and is very bad for you and costs 100 dollars, and we had to buy it for 3 months. (AS)

Another factor affecting affordability were the long waiting times for public services. Both AR and AP—a migrant from a Western non-European country—highlighted the significant purchasing power required to access private sexual health services when public services are overburdened.

> The sexual health (…) you can go privately if you have the money. If you have an STD or something you have to take care of yourself (…) You have to go private in the end because the public doesn't really seem to exist. Like, again once you can, you can go private and see someone quickly. (AP)
> Other way you can go to private and pay hundreds of euro to get tested. (AR)

Adding another layer of complexity, LA—a migrant sex worker from Latin America—delved into the unpredictability of affordability, which is particularly pertinent for individuals engaged in sex work and other forms of precarious work.

> I asked the doctor to get a gynaecologist and it was like in January and like my appointment is in June. (…) For routine, you know, once a year that we need to do it, and so it's in June. So if I want to get it soon I need to pay extra, for this special test. So yeah, I think it's very vulnerable. I can pay it but it's not like I can pay it every month, you know? (LA)

Findings indicated that participants acknowledged a satisfactory level of service affordability, with Malta being commended for providing free public sexual health services. However, financial challenges were noted, stemming from the need to access private services due to lengthy waiting times in the public sector and the cost of HIV treatment for those without a residence permit. Income fluctuations, a characteristic feature of precarious work, were highlighted as a significant factor influencing affordability.

4.5.5 Appropriateness

Appropriateness speaks to the match between the offer made by services and clients' needs, including in terms of timing/timeliness, technical and interpersonal quality of services and coordination between different offices/departments. This

[4]Since 2025, the Malta GU Clinic updated its HIV treatment requirements: one month's payslip (instead of multiple payslips) is now needed.

dimension also concerns itself with individuals' empowerment and ability to engage in care (Levesque et al. 2013).

The saturation of public sexual health services on the island was again identified as a key factor affecting timeliness and, by extension, appropriateness. AR and AP highlighted how delays hinder patients' ability to secure appointments, including for preventive care.

> the queues to get into STD tests is half year, 9 months to get into if you are symptomless. (AR)
> I called one time, 'I want an STD test' and they were like, 'Yeah, we have a spot for you in three months'. Like, what the hell?! Like, this is a joke. How is this going to protect anyone if the only time you can get a free STD test, you know, is once in the future after you have already infected a bunch of people?!(AP)

Participants' ability to consistently engage in care—such as adhering to health professionals' advice on safe sexual practices, testing frequency, or treatment—varied. For instance, LO, quoted earlier in this chapter, found adherence to HIV treatment straightforward due to his strong awareness of the importance of self-care. Conversely, AS, a migrant from Latin America, spoke with a blend of pride and frustration about the caregiving role he naturally assumed within his small sex-working community:

> We're 9 in total and those are the girls I take to the sexual health clinic because we're working and we need to get tested. Most clients want oral sex without a condom and we need prep. I take all of them to the clinic (…) But then [name of partner] is very lazy. If I didn't do it, he wouldn't. (AS)

AS also reflected on his role within his sex-working community when responding to an incident of violence, further highlighting gaps in service coordination. Recounting an episode in which he called the police after a fellow sex worker was nearly fatally strangled by a client, AS expressed deep dismay at the authorities' complete failure to provide support. This failure extended not only to ensuring access to rights but also to offering referrals for healthcare.

> And the police: 'We can't do anything for you'. If you know the person's name, then you can report him, otherwise nothing. I told them, 'Look—they need to go to hospital to get a check-up.' They did not tell us, Yeah, look, this is the phone number that you can call in these cases to ask for help, or if it's urgent, the police won't say no, this is the number'. Nope. The police told us, "It's your problem, since you're doing this [sex work], you have to deal with it. (AS)

Having to "deal with it" on their own thus emerges as a defining aspect of both local and migrant sex workers' management of violence in a context where sex work is criminalised. In terms of the appropriateness of sexual health services for migrant sex workers, based on the insights gleaned from participants, this appears to be largely influenced by gaps in timeliness, and lack of coordination between public services, particularly concerning in cases of violence.

4.6 What Next?

The findings in this chapter highlight the significant challenges faced by many migrant sex workers in accessing sexual health services in Malta, including after experiences of violence. The primary obstacles identified fall within the dimensions of acceptability, availability, accommodation and affordability, with additional concerns raised regarding appropriateness. Barriers such as strict residency and taxation requirements for HIV treatment, as well as the reliance on private healthcare due to delays in public sexual health services, remain particularly problematic. However, the government's recent efforts to decentralise sexual health services, including the introduction of a mobile unit targeting key populations, are expected to help address these issues significantly (National Sexual Health Strategy Malta 2024).

The analysis of acceptability revealed significant concerns, particularly regarding the impact of intersecting gender, sex-work, and race-related biases among practitioners on access to dignified care, especially in cases of sexual and other violence experienced during sex work. This dimension presented as being strongly impacted by prevailing beliefs about women's bodies, and more broadly, the bodies and rights of sex workers. While not the primary focus of this chapter, these biases are not limited to healthcare providers but extend to the police and society at large, as evidenced by the discussion on appropriateness and corroborated by numerous participants. This societal context significantly undermines sex workers' ability to access timely and dignified healthcare and rights. When gender intersects with precarious migrant status, violence may often remain hidden, as fear of repercussions deters migrant sex workers from seeking help or speaking out.

In line with international research speaking to the importance of decriminalisation for positive sexual health outcomes for sex workers, the authors emphasise the need to move beyond restrictive policy arrangements on sex work that negatively impact sex workers' health (Grenfell et al. 2023; Oliveira et al. 2023; Johnson et al. 2023). Furthermore, they call on the Maltese government to improve access to HIV treatment for those who require it, thereby aligning more closely with European and international human rights standards (De Vito et al. 2016; Stefano 2022). Specific training for healthcare providers on working with migrant sex workers, along with the co-development and co-delivery of services, would significantly improve access to care (Johnson et al. 2023).

This chapter underscored the importance of moving beyond stereotypical portrayals of migrants and sex workers as "disease-carriers." Participants in the study demonstrated awareness and a general sense of responsibility regarding prevention and self-care. While this may not represent the entire migrant or sex-working population, positive examples of self-organisation to ensure access to sexual healthcare highlight the value of peer education and mutual support. Future research should further investigate the role of peer education, aiming to build a stronger evidence base for targeted interventions. Similarly, future research should also consider exploring sex worker-led strategies which can contribute towards behavioural change in governmental institutions such as healthcare or law enforcement (Rao Biradavolu et al. 2009).

Currently, research on sex work in Malta remains limited. More in-depth studies are needed to fully understand the experiences of migrant sex workers and to explore the challenges healthcare professionals face in addressing their needs. Such research will be greatly facilitated by a legal and policy framework that decriminalises sex work, creating a more supportive environment for both service users and providers.

Finally, this chapter underscores the critical importance of fostering collaboration and data-sharing among researchers, policymakers, and service providers to build a robust evidence base on sex work in Malta. By comparing and integrating diverse data sets, as the authors have done here and elsewhere (Camilleri and Rossoni 2026), stakeholders can uncover deeper insights into the needs, challenges, and lived experiences of sex workers. The authors emphasise that such collaborative efforts are essential not only for advancing knowledge but also for informing evidence-driven policies and interventions that promote the dignity, rights, and well-being of sex workers. They strongly encourage similar forms of partnership as a foundation for meaningful change and improved outcomes across sectors.

References

Albright E, D'Adamo K (2017) Decreasing human trafficking through sex work decriminalization. AMA J Ethics 19(1):123

Atkinson R, Flint J (2011) Sampling, snowball: accessing hidden and hard-to-reach populations. In: Miller RL, Brewer J (eds) The A-Z of social research. SAGE Publications Ltd, London, pp 275–280

Benoit C, Jansson M, Smith M, Flagg J (2018) Prostitution stigma and its effect on the working conditions, personal lives, and health of sex workers. J Sex Res 55(4–5):457–471. https://doi.org/10.1080/00224499.2017.1393652

Calderaro C, Giametta C (2019) "The problem of prostitution": repressive Policies in the Name of Migration Control, Public Order, and Women's Rights in France. Anti-Trafficking Rev 12:155–171. https://doi.org/10.14197/atr.2012191210

Camilleri J (2025) Choices, boundaries, and ideological divides: a study of sex work in Malta. UCL. https://discovery.ucl.ac.uk/id/eprint/10209494/

Camilleri J, Rossoni I (2026) Charting sex work in malta: first steps. Sociol Res Online. https://doi.org/10.1177/13607804261421049.

Camilleri J, Cockbain E, Belur J (2025) Reframing research participation as labour: lessons from sex work research. Int J Qual Methods 24. https://doi.org/10.1177/16094069251409618./p

Crumb L, Mingo TM, Crowe A (2019) 'Get over it and move on': the impact of mental illness stigma in rural, low-income United States populations. Ment Health Prev 13:143–148. https://doi.org/10.1016/j.mhp.2019.01.010

De Vito E, de Waure C, Specchia ML, Parente P, Azzolini E, Frisicale EM, Favale M, Teleman AA, Ricciardi W (2016) Are undocumented Migrants' entitlements and barriers to healthcare a public health challenge for the European Union? Public Health Rev 37(1):13. https://doi.org/10.1186/s40985-016-0026-3

Deering KN, Amin A, Shoveller J, Nesbitt A, Garcia-Moreno C, Duff P, Argento E, Shannon K (2014) A systematic review of the correlates of violence against sex workers. Am J Public Health 104(5):e42–e54. https://doi.org/10.2105/AJPH.2014.301909

Elgabry M, Camilleri J (2021) Conducting hidden populations research: a reflective case study on researching the Biohacking community. Futures 132(102769):5. https://doi.org/10.1016/j.futures.2021.102769

Elmir E, Schmied V, Jackson D, Wilkes L (2011) Interviewing people about potentially sensitive topics. Nurse Res 19(1):12–16

ESWA Applauds the Position of the UN Working Group on Discrimination against Women and Girls (2025) European Sex Workers' Rights Alliance. https://www.eswalliance.org/eswa_applauds_eliminating_discrimination_against_sx_workers_securing_their_human_rights. Accessed 2 Jan 2024

Faissner M, Beckmann L, Freistein K, Jungilligens K, Braun E (2024) Healthcare for sex workers—access, barriers, and needs: an exploratory qualitative interview study. Ethik Med 36(2):151–168. https://doi.org/10.1007/s00481-024-00815-8

Farley M (1994) Prostitution: the oldest use and abuse of women. Off Our Backs 24(5):14–22

Faugier J, Sargeant M (1997) Sampling hard to reach populations. J Adv Nurs 26:790–797

Goldenberg SM, Thomas RM, Forbes A, Baral S (2021) Overview and evidence-based recommendations to address health and human rights inequities faced by sex workers. In: Goldenberg SM, Thomas RM, Forbes A, Baral S (eds) Sex work, health, and human rights: global inequities, challenges, and opportunities. Springer, Cham. http://www.ncbi.nlm.nih.gov/books/NBK585700/

Government of Malta (2007) Chapter 63 – White Slave Traffic (Suppression) Ordinance. https://legislation.mt/eli/cap/63/eng/pdf

Government of Malta (2019) Reform on human trafficking and prostitution - public consultation document (Valletta, Malta)

Government of Malta (2024a) Chapter 16 – Civil Code, pt. 1618, https://legislation.mt/eli/cap/16/20241025/eng

Government of Malta (2024b) Chapter 9 – Criminal Code, pts. 197, 204 and 205, https://legislation.mt/eli/cap/9/20241025/eng

Government of Malta (n.d.) Chapter 16 – Civil Code, pts. 251, 623 and 1618

Grenfell, P, Stuart, R, Eastham, J, Gallagher, A, Elmes, J, Platt, L and O'Neill, M (2023) Policing and public health interventions into sex workers' lives: necropolitical assemblages and alternative visions of social justice. Crit Public Health 33(3):282–296. https://doi.org/10.1080/09581596.2022.2096428

Guest G, Namey EE, Mitchell ML (2013) In-depth interviews in collecting qualitative data: a field manual for applied research. SAGE Publications, Ltd, London, pp 113–171. https://doi.org/10.4135/9781506374680

Head E (2009) The ethics and implications of paying participants in qualitative research. Int J Soc Res Methodol 12(4):335–344. https://doi.org/10.1080/13645570802246724

Heaton J (2022) Pseudonyms are used throughout: a footnote. Unpacked Qual Inq 28(1):123–132. https://doi.org/10.1177/10778004211048379

Heckathorn DD (1997a) Respondent-driven sampling: a new approach to the study of hidden populations. Soc Probl 44(2):174

Heckathorn DD (1997b) Respondent-driven sampling II: deriving valid population estimates from chain-referral samples of hidden populations. Soc Probl 49(1):11

Hughes DM (2000) The "Natasha" trade: the transnational shadow market of trafficking in women. J Int Aff 53(2):625–651

International Women's Rights Action Watch Asia Pacific (2017) Framework on Rights of Sex Workers & CEDAW. https://law.yale.edu/sites/default/files/area/center/ghjp/documents/framework_on_rights_of_sex_workers_cedaw.pdf

Jansson M, Smith M, Benoit C, Magnuson D, Healey P (2023) Challenges and benefits of disclosure of sex work to intimate partners. J Sex Res 60(6):890–902. https://doi.org/10.1080/00224499.2022.2092587

Johnson L, Potter LC, Beeching H, Bradbury M, Matos B, Sumner S, Wills L et al (2023) Interventions to improve health and the determinants of health among sex workers in high-income countries: a systematic review. Lancet Public Health 8(2):e141–e154. https://doi.org/10.1016/S2468-2667(22)00252-3

Kada R (2019) Cultural adaptations of CBT for the British Jewish orthodox community. Cog Behav Ther 12:1–9. https://doi.org/10.1017/S1754470X18000120

King N, Horrocks C, Brooks J (2019) Interviews in qualitative research, 2nd edn. SAGE Publications

Kloek M, De Vlas SJ, Hontelez JAC (2024) High rates of violence and low police reporting amongst sex Workers in The Netherlands during the COVID-19 pandemic. Crime Sci 13(1):38. https://doi.org/10.1186/s40163-024-00237-3

Krüsi A, Pacey K, Bird L, Taylor C, Chettiar K, Allan S, Bennett D, Montaner JS, Kerr T, Shannon K (2014) Criminalisation of clients: reproducing vulnerabilities for violence and poor health among street-based sex Workers in Canada – a qualitative study. BMJ Open 4(6):1–10. https://doi.org/10.1136/bmjopen-2014-005191>

Lawan UM, Abubakar S, Ahmed A (2012) Risk perceptions, prevention and treatment seeking for sexually transmitted infections and HIV/AIDS among female sex Workers in Kano, Nigeria. Afr J Reprod Health 16(1):61–67

Lazarus L, Deering KN, Nabees R, Gibson K, Tyndall MW, Shannon k (2012) Occupational stigma as a primary barrier to health Care for street-based sex workers in Canada. Cult Health Sex 14(2):39–50. https://doi.org/10.1080/13691058.2011.628411

Levesque J-F, Harris MF, Russell G (2013) Patient-CENTRED access to health care: conceptualising access at the interface of health systems and populations. Int J Equity Health 12(1):18. https://doi.org/10.1186/1475-9276-12-18

Li Y (2011) Translating interviews, translating lives: ethical considerations in cross-language narrative Inquiry. TESL Can J 16(30.5):16–30

Liu M (2012) Chinese migrant women in the sex industry: exploring their paths to prostitution. Fem Criminol 7(4):327–349. https://doi.org/10.1177/1557085112436836

Lynzi A (2019) Stigma, decriminalisation, and violence against street-based sex workers: changing the narrative. Sexualities 22(7–8):1288–1308. https://doi.org/10.1177/1363460718780216

McBride B, Janushev T (2021) Criminalisation, health, and labour rights among Im/migrant sex workers globally'. In: Goldenberg SM, Morgan Thomas R, Forbes A, Baral B (eds) Sex work, health, and human rights: global inequities, challenges, and opportunities for action. Springer, Cham. http://www.ncbi.nlm.nih.gov/books/NBK585685/

McBride B, Shannon K, Bingham B, Braschel M, Strathdee S, Goldenberg SM (2020) Underreporting of violence to police among women sex workers in Canada: amplified inequities for Im/migrant and in-call workers prior to and following end-demand legislation. Health Hum Rights J 22(2):257–270

Modupe-Oluwa BE, Heumann S (2014) Migration, sex work and exploitative labor conditions: experiences of Nigerian Women in the Sex Industry in Turin, Italy, and counter-trafficking measures. Gender Technol Dev 18(1):77–105. https://doi.org/10.1177/0971852413515322

Moen OM (2014) Is prostitution harmful? J Med Ethics 40(2):73

Monique Agius (2022) Four women plead guilty to participating in running of Gżira brothel, Newsbook Malta. https://newsbook.com.mt/en/four-women-plead-guilty-to-participating-in-running-of-gzira-brothel. Accessed 2 Jan 2024

Monique Agius (2023) Two women admit using their apartment for prostitution, Newsbook Malta. https://newsbook.com.mt/en/two-women-admit-using-their-apartment-for-prostitution. Accessed 2 Jan 2024

National Sexual Health Strategy Malta (2024). Retrieved from: https://health.gov.mt/wp-content/uploads/2024/12/National_Sexual_Health_Strategy_2025_2030.pdf

Nussbaum MN (1998) Whether from reason or prejudice: taking money for bodily services. J Leg Stud 27(S2):707

Oliveira A, Lemos A, Mota M, Pinto R (2023) Understanding the impact of EU prostitution policies on sex workers: a mixed study systematic review. Sex Res Soc Policy 20(4):1448–1468. https://doi.org/10.1007/s13178-023-00814-2

Padovese V, Farrugia S, Almabrok Ali Ghat S, Rossoni I (2021) Sexually transmitted infections' epidemiology and knowledge, attitude and practice survey in a set of migrants attending the sexual health Clinic in Malta. J Eur Acad Dermatol Venereol 35(2):509–516. https://doi.org/10.1111/jdv.16949

Rossoni I, Chollier M, Dudushi R, Ghigo J, Padovese V (2023) A scoping review of sexual and reproductive health recommendations in the context of migration to Europe. J Eur Acad Dermatol Venereol 37(12):2450–2461. https://doi.org/10.1111/jdv.19428

Oriol M, Padovese V, Folch C, Rossoni I, Marks M, Rodríguez MA, Arias I, Telenti A et al (2023) Epidemiology and Determinants of Reemerging Bacterial Sexually Transmitted Infections (STIs) and Emerging STIs in Europe. Lancet Region Health – Eur 34:100742. https://doi.org/10.1016/j.lanepe.2023.100742

Penfold C, Hunter G, Campbell R, Barham L (2004) Tackling client violence in female street prostitution: inter-agency working between outreach agencies and the Police. Policing Soc 14(4):365–379. https://doi.org/10.1080/1043946042000286074

Platt L, Grenfell P, Meiksin R, Elmes J, Sherman SG, Sanders T, Mwangi P, Crago AL (2018) Associations between sex work laws and sex workers' health: a systematic review and meta-analysis of quantitative and qualitative studies. PLoS Med. https://doi.org/10.1371/journal.pmed.1002680

Rao Biradavolu M, Burris S, George A, Jena A, Blankenship KM (2009) Can sex workers regulate police? Learning from an HIV prevention project for sex workers in Southern India. Soc Sci Med 68(8):1541–1544. https://doi.org/10.1016/j.socscimed.2009.01.040

Raymond J (2003) Ten reasons for not legalizing prostitution and a legal response to the demand for prostitution. J Trauma Pract 2:315–332

Raymond J (2013) Myths and mythmakers of prostitution in not a choice, not a job. University of Nebraska Press, Potomac Books, Nebraska, pp 1–36

Ripley EDB (2006) A review of paying research participants: it's time to move beyond the ethical debate. J Empir Res Hum Ethics 1(4):9–20. https://doi.org/10.1525/jer.2006.1.4.9
Rita H, Öztürk B, Foverskov E, Pedersen L, Sørensen HT, Bøtker HE et al (2022) Migrants' health and persisting barriers to accessing health-care systems. EClinMed 44:101321. https://doi.org/10.1016/j.eclinm.2022.101321
Rocha-Jiménez T, Brouwer KC, Silverman JG, Morales-Miranda S, Goldenberg SM (2016) Migration, violence, and Safety among migrant sex workers: a qualitative study in two guatemalan communities. culture. Health Sex 18(9):965–979. https://doi.org/10.1080/13691058.2015.1122229
Rosie C, Smith L, Leacy B, Ryan M, Stoica B (2020) Not collateral damage: trends in violence and hate crimes experienced by sex workers in the Republic of Ireland. Irish J Sociol: IJS 28(3):280–313. https://doi.org/10.1177/0791603520939794
Rossoni I (2026a) Crafting vulneramentality: Vulnerability (and resistance) among migrants with experiences of sex work in Malta. Eur J Criminol. https://doi.org/10.1177/14773708251400844
Rossoni I (2026b) Manufacturing Vulnerability: Sex Work, Migration, and Trafficking on the Southern Borders of Europe. Leiden University. https://hdl.handle.net/1887/4297578
Rossoni I, Van der Woude, M (2025) 'Resisting "Manufactured" vulnerability: discretionary policing and migrant sex workers' Resistance Strategies in Malta', Int J Crime Justice Soc Democr. https://doi.org/10.5204/ijcjsd.3909.
Rossoni I, Gauci D, Gauci Farrugia S, Padovese V (2022) Gender, migration and violence among third country nationals accessing the sexual health clinic in Malta. J Eur Acad Dermatol Venereol 36(9):1623–1631. https://doi.org/10.1111/jdv.18222
Sampethai V (2022) Workers, migrants, and queers: the political economy of community among illegalised sex workers in Athens. Anti-Trafficking Rev 19:28–46. https://doi.org/10.14197/atr.201222193
Scicluna P, Clark M (2019) Victimisation and addictive careers amongst women in Malta. J Forensic Pract 21(1):71–84. https://doi.org/10.1108/JFP-07-2018-0031
Shaver FM (2005) Sex work research: methodological and ethical challenges. J Interpers Violence 20(3):296–319. https://doi.org/10.1177/0886260504274340
Ślęzak I (2018) Research on indoor sex work in Poland: An Ethnographer's dilemmas. Oñati Socio-Legal Ser 8(8):1134–1150. https://doi.org/10.35295/osls.iisl/0000-0000-0000-0988
Smith M, Mac J (2018) Revolting prostitutes, vol 1. Verso, London
Stefano A (2022) The right to health care of irregular migrants: between primary care and emergency treatment in irregular migrants and the right to health. Cambridge University Press, Cambridge. https://doi.org/10.1017/9781009051750.005
Struyf P (2023) To report or not to report? A systematic review of sex workers' willingness to report violence and victimization to police. Trauma Violence Abuse 24(5):3065–3077. https://doi.org/10.1177/15248380221122819
SWERV: Sex Workers Evaluate Reporting Violence—National Ugly Mugs. https://nationaluglymugs.org/swerv-sex-workers-evaluate-reporting-violence/. Accessed 2 Jan 2025
Thomas RM (2021) Conflation of sex work and trafficking' (NSWP – Global Network of Sex Work Projects). https://www.nswp.org/sites/default/files/nswp_written_statement_-_hlm_on_trafficking_in_persons_november_2021.pdf
Turcotte M, Lanctôt N (2021) Managing the toll of sex work with bounded agency: perspectives of ex-sex workers. Can J Hum Sex 30(3):296–305. https://doi.org/10.3138/CJHS.2020-0030
Vanwesenbeeck I (2017) Sex work criminalization is barking up the wrong tree. Arch Sex Behav 46(6):1632. https://doi.org/10.1007/s10508-017-1008-3
Vuolajärvi N (2019) Precarious intimacies—Europeanised border regime and migrant sex work. J Ethn Migr Stud 45(7):1090–1107. https://doi.org/10.1080/1369183X.2018.1430558
Weitzer R (2012) Sex trafficking and the sex industry: the need for evidence-based theory and legislation. J Crim Law Criminol 101(4):1337–1369
Wiebel WW (1998) Identifying and gaining access to hidden populations. In: Lambert EY (ed) The collection and interpretation of data from hidden populations. U.S. Department of Health and Human Services, Rockville, p 6
Zhang SX, Spiller MW, Finch BK, Qin Y (2014) Estimating labor trafficking among unauthorized migrant workers in San Diego. Ann Am Acad Pol Soc Sci 653(1):65–86. https://doi.org/10.1177/0002716213519237

5 Conflict, Internal Displacement, and Sexual Health: An African Experience

Wendemagegn Enbiale

Contents

Abstract

This chapter aims to examine the intersection of conflict, displacement, and sexual health in Africa, highlighting existing gaps, policy challenges, and opportunities for intervention. More specifically, it delves deeper into challenges related to sexually transmitted infections (STIs), HIV in humanitarian settings, sexual violence (SV), and, more broadly, gender-based violence (GBV). By shedding light on these complex and interlocking issues, the chapter advocates for a more inclusive, rights-based approach that prioritizes the sexual and reproductive health of displaced populations in Africa.

W. Enbiale (✉)
Department of Dermatovenereology, College of Medicine and Health Sciences, Bahir Dar University, Bahir Dar, Ethiopia

Collaborative Research and Training Center for Neglected Tropical Diseases, Arba Minch University, Arba Minch, Ethiopia

V. Padovese, I. Rossoni (eds.), *Intersections of Sexual Health, Migration and Sexualised Violence*, Sustainable Development Goals Series, https://doi.org/10.1007/978-3-032-20707-4_5

Keywords

Internal displacement · Conflict · STIs · HIV · Sexual health · GBV · Africa

5.1 Introduction

Africa is home to one of the world's largest internally displaced populations (IDPs) due to protracted conflicts, political instability, and climate-related disasters. As of 2023, more than 35 million people were internally displaced from conflict across the continent, representing nearly half of the global total. Floods and droughts are also another major contributor to IDP in Africa, and the number has risen nearly sixfold across the continent in the last 15 years, from 1.1 million in 2009 to 6.3 million in 2023. Conflict remains the primary driver of displacement; five countries such as Sudan, the Democratic Republic of the Congo (DRC), Somalia, Nigeria, and Ethiopia represent about 80% of the IDPs by conflict or violence in Africa (Internal Displacement Monitoring Centre (IDMC) 2023a). And also, East Africa has been the scene of some of the world's largest conflict displacement crises, including Ethiopia's Tigray and Amhara regions and, more recently, Sudan. Other countries such as DRC, Somalia, and South Sudan have also experienced protracted conflict and displacement (Arage et al. 2023; Tsadik et al. 2024; Mohamed 2025; Kavulikirwa 2024).

Internal displacement disrupts social structures, economic stability, and healthcare systems, making already vulnerable populations—particularly women and girls—more susceptible to sexual and reproductive health challenges (Fiedler 2023; Vesco et al. 2025; Dafallah et al. 2023). The consequences of displacement extend beyond immediate survival, as it increases exposure to gender-based violence (GBV), limited access to contraceptive services, unsafe abortions, sexually transmitted infections (STIs) including HIV, and maternal health risks (Tewabe et al. 2024; Tol et al. 2013; Murphy et al. 2023; World Health Organization 2020).

Displaced women and girls face unique sexual health challenges that are often overlooked in humanitarian responses. Studies show that more than 60% of preventable maternal deaths, 53% of under-five deaths, and 45% of neonatal deaths occur in conflict and displacement settings (World Health Organization 2020). The breakdown of healthcare services, lack of privacy in overcrowded IDP camps, and inadequate access to contraception lead to increased rates of unintended pregnancies, unsafe abortions, and complications during childbirth (International Planned Parenthood Federation n.d.).

Moreover, sexual violence is rampant in displacement settings, with armed groups and opportunistic perpetrators exploiting the vulnerability of displaced women. The 2023 report highlights a 50% increase in conflict-related sexual violence compared to the previous year, with 3688 UN-verified cases recorded across 21 conflict zones. This surge is particularly concerning given the severe restrictions on humanitarian access worldwide (United Nations 2024a). Many survivors lack access to post-exposure prophylaxis (PEP), emergency contraception, and psychological support, further exacerbating their trauma. Cultural barriers and stigmatization of survivors also deter women from seeking care, deepening the cycle of neglect and health deterioration (World Health Organization 2020).

Despite international frameworks such as the African Union's Kampala Convention (2009)—which aims to protect IDPs and ensure their rights—implementation remains inconsistent (United Nations Office for the Coordination of Humanitarian Affairs (OCHA) 2004; African Union's (Kampala Convention) 2009). The lack of government accountability, insufficient funding, and weak health infrastructure in many African countries has left displaced populations without adequate reproductive health services (World Health Organization 2020; Adeola 2021; Kelly 2021).

Key barriers include:

- Limited access to contraception: IDP women are twice as likely to have an unmet need for family planning compared to non-displaced populations.

- Lack of skilled birth attendants: Many IDP camps lack trained midwives and obstetricians, leading to high maternal and neonatal mortality.
- Inadequate sexual violence response: Few healthcare facilities provide integrated GBV services, and many survivors remain unprotected and untreated.

While humanitarian organizations have provided temporary relief through mobile clinics and outreach services, long-term strategies are needed to integrate sexual and reproductive health (SRH) into national health policies and IDP response frameworks. Strengthening health systems, ensuring legal protections for displaced women, and promoting sexual health education are critical steps towards addressing this crisis (World Health Organization 2020).

5.2 Sexually Transmitted Infections (STIs) in Displacement Settings: Challenges and Responses

5.2.1 Prevalence and Risk Factors During Displacement

Displacement due to conflict, natural disasters, and political instability places populations at heightened risk for sexually transmitted infections (STIs). But studies on the prevalence of STIs in refugee camps are very scarce; most of the data available are derived from medical campaigns and refugee clinics. A study conducted across 15 sub-Saharan African countries found that women who experienced sexual violence in the past 12 months were 1.76 times more likely to self-report sexually transmitted infections (STIs) compared to those who did not experience such violence (adjusted odds ratio [aOR] = 1.76, 95% confidence interval [CI] = 1.59–1.94) (Aboagye et al. 2023; United Nations Population Fund 2023). This finding suggests a higher prevalence of STIs among displaced populations, who are often at increased risk of sexual violence. A UNFPA report from a camp in North Kivu Province, The Democratic Republic of the Congo, states that in less than 2 months, out of 3000 displaced people, 200 have diagnosed with sexually transmitted diseases (Siraw et al. 2019). A cross-sectional study on refugees from Eritrea, Somalia, and South Sudan has found the overall prevalence of symptomatic sexually transmitted diseases was 34.6% (95%CI: 29.8%, 39.6%) (Kim et al. 2009). A comparative study between undisplaced populations and IDPs in DRC showed that women living in IDP camps in DRC were shown to have four times the rates of STI compared to host populations, which is associated with conflict-related sexual violence and unprotected sex (Kidie et al. 2025).

The breakdown of health infrastructure during displacement further contributes to increased STI transmission. With healthcare services disrupted, routine STI screenings, preventive interventions, and treatment programmes become inaccessible. This lack of medical services is particularly detrimental to displaced women, who face a high risk of sexual exploitation and gender-based violence (World Health Organization 2020). The situation in Ethiopia's conflict-affected areas, for example, has shown that widespread sexual violence is a driver of increased STI transmission, highlighting the urgent need for targeted interventions (United Nations Population Fund 2023; Fahme et al. 2024).

Another contributing factor is the socioeconomic vulnerability of displaced individuals. Many engage in transactional sex for survival, increasing their risk of exposure to STIs. Studies from Africa's refugee camps show that young women, in particular, are coerced into sex in exchange for food, security, or shelter, often without access to condoms or other protective measures (Mayaud et al. 1997). The risk is further compounded by overcrowded and insecure living conditions in IDP camps, where privacy is limited, and women and girls face heightened exposure to sexual coercion (Moffa et al. 2025). A recent publication from Uganda has shown that migrants exhibited a significantly higher combined prevalence of curable STIs (gonorrhoea, chlamydia, high-titre syphilis (rapid plasma regain ≥1:8) and trichomoniasis) as compared with long-term residents (34.4% vs 24.2%; adjPRR = 1.23; 95% CI 1.03 to 1.47) (Vasylyeva et al. 2022).

5.2.1.1 Barriers to STI Prevention and Access to Testing

Access to STI prevention, testing, and treatment services remains a significant challenge in displacement settings. Humanitarian crises often disrupt healthcare supply chains, making essential STI prevention tools such as condoms, pre-exposure prophylaxis (PrEP), and post-exposure prophylaxis (PEP) unavailable (Kvasnevska et al. 2024). In war-torn regions like Ukraine, research has shown that limited access to contraception and sexual health services during displacement has led to a surge in STI cases (Okorafor et al. 2024).

Another critical barrier is the lack of trained healthcare workers in conflict-affected areas. Many clinicians flee during crises, leaving displaced populations without skilled personnel to diagnose and manage STIs. This lack of expertise leads to delayed diagnoses and untreated infections, increasing the likelihood of complications and onward transmission. Moreover, the stigma surrounding STIs discourages individuals from seeking care. In many African cultures, STI diagnosis carries social shame, which prevents individuals from disclosing symptoms or accessing health services, especially in displacement settings where privacy is scarce (Kvasnevska et al. 2024; Desrosiers et al. 2020).

The lack of community-based education programmes also hinders STI prevention efforts. In stable settings, awareness campaigns promote condom use, STI screening, and safe sexual practices. However, during displacement, these initiatives are often deprioritized in favour of more immediate humanitarian needs such as food and shelter. Consequently, many displaced individuals lack the knowledge to protect themselves from STIs or recognize symptoms early (World Health Organization 2021).

5.2.1.2 Syndromic Management of STIs (WHO) and Its Limitations

The World Health Organization (WHO) recommends syndromic management as the primary STI treatment approach in resource-limited settings, including displacement camps. This strategy involves diagnosing and treating STIs based on symptoms rather than laboratory tests, allowing healthcare providers to administer treatment even when diagnostic facilities are unavailable. Given the challenges of laboratory access in conflict zones, syndromic management is often the only feasible option for addressing STIs among displaced populations (Padovese and Knapp 2021).

While syndromic management is useful in humanitarian crises, it has notable limitations. First, many STIs are asymptomatic, meaning infected individuals who do not show symptoms go untreated, leading to continued transmission. Research from IDP camps in Africa has shown that a significant proportion of individuals with gonorrhoea and chlamydia infections do not exhibit symptoms, which means syndromic management alone is insufficient for comprehensive STI control (Chen et al. 2008; White et al. 2008; van der Eem et al. 2016; Otieno et al. 2014). Another limitation is the potential for misdiagnosis and overtreatment. Syndromic management relies on clinical symptoms that can overlap with non-STI conditions, leading to incorrect treatments and unnecessary use of antibiotics. This approach contributes to antimicrobial resistance, particularly for infections like gonorrhoea, where antibiotic resistance is a growing concern globally. Additionally, syndromic management does not account for co-infections, which are common among displaced populations exposed to multiple risk factors (Gupta and Sharma 2019; Holt et al. 2003).

Despite these limitations, syndromic management remains a crucial intervention in displacement settings where diagnostic infrastructure is lacking. To improve its effectiveness, humanitarian agencies must integrate STI testing into broader health programmes and advocate for rapid diagnostic tools that can be deployed in crisis settings. Mobile health clinics and community-based outreach services can also help bridge gaps in STI care by bringing services directly to affected populations (Morris 2009; Amodu et al. 2020).

In conclusion, STIs remain a critical yet under-addressed public health challenge in displacement settings, where conflict, insecurity, and economic vulnerability create conditions for increased transmission. While syndromic management provides an immediate response in crisis settings, it should be complemented with broader strategies that include expanded testing, improved access to STI prevention tools, and strengthened community education programmes. Addressing STIs in displacement settings requires a multisectoral approach, integrating sexual health services into humanitarian responses while ensuring that displaced individuals have access to the care and protection they need (Amodu et al. 2020).

- To reduce STI transmission and improve health outcomes, international organizations, governments, and humanitarian actors must prioritize:
- Increasing STI screening and diagnostic capacity in refugee and IDP camps to move beyond symptom-based treatment.
- Ensuring a steady supply of STI prevention resources, including condoms, PrEP, and PEP, in humanitarian aid packages.
- Expanding access to STI treatment through mobile clinics and community-based healthcare models in displacement settings.
- Integrating gender-based violence response services with STI care to support survivors of sexual violence.
- Strengthening health education programmes to promote safer sexual practices and reduce stigma around STI treatment.

5.3 HIV in Conflict-Affected Populations in Africa: Challenges and Responses

5.3.1 HIV Burden and Risks for Conflict-Affected Populations

Armed conflict and forced displacement significantly heighten the risk of HIV transmission and poor health outcomes among affected populations in Africa. The continent hosts the largest number of internally displaced persons (IDPs), exacerbating already fragile healthcare systems and leading to gaps in HIV prevention, treatment, and care (Boeyink et al. 2022). Studies indicate that displaced populations often experience higher HIV prevalence than non-displaced communities due to several interconnected factors, including the breakdown of healthcare services, increased sexual violence, and the disruption of social support networks (Dellie et al. 2024).

Women living in IDP camps in the Democratic Republic of Congo (DRC) were found to have twice the rates of HIV compared to host populations, largely due to conflict-related sexual violence and lack of protective interventions (Ouma et al. 2021). The intersection of conflict and HIV risk is particularly evident in war-torn regions such as South Sudan, the DRC, and parts of the Sahel, where instability has severely weakened public health responses (Kodo et al. 2024). Forced migration further increases exposure to high-risk sexual behaviour, as individuals are often placed in overcrowded and insecure environments where exploitation and transactional sex become survival strategies (https://www.amnesty.org/en/latest/news/2022/02/ethiopia-tigrayan-forces-murder-rape-and-pillage-in-attacks-on-civilians-in-amhara-towns/ n.d.). In some refugee and IDP camps in Africa, HIV incidence rates are significantly higher than in surrounding host communities due to the absence of structured prevention programmes and strained local healthcare systems (Mesfin et al. 2023).

5.4 Disruption of HIV Prevention Programmes

HIV prevention programmes are among the first casualties in conflict zones, leading to increased transmission rates among vulnerable populations. The collapse of health infrastructure and displacement of medical personnel hinder the availability of essential services such as voluntary counselling and testing (VCT), condom distribution, pre-exposure prophylaxis (PrEP), and harm reduction programmes (Boeyink et al. 2022). The discontinuation of these interventions leaves large portions of displaced populations unprotected from new infections.

A major challenge in conflict settings is the breakdown of supply chains, preventing essential commodities like condoms and PrEP from reaching those in need (Ouma et al. 2021). This results in individuals engaging in unprotected sex due to the unavailability of protective measures. The loss of community-based education programmes further worsens the problem, as awareness campaigns that promote safe sexual practices and HIV risk reduction are often halted due to conflict-related instability (Workie et al. 2023).

Sexual violence in conflict settings further exacerbates the HIV epidemic. Reports from Ethiopia, the Central African Republic, and northern Nigeria reveal that armed groups have used rape as a weapon of war, increasing HIV exposure among survivors who often lack access to post-exposure prophylaxis (PEP) or emergency healthcare services (Kodo et al. 2024; Internal Displacement Monitoring Centre (IDMC) 2023a). Another critical challenge is the disruption of maternal and child health services, including the prevention of mother-to-child transmission (PMTCT) programmes. In conflict zones, pregnant women living with HIV often lose access to critical antenatal care services, increasing the risk of perinatal HIV transmission (https://www.amnesty.org/en/latest/news/2022/02/ethiopia-tigrayan-forces-murder-rape-and-pillage-in-attacks-on-civilians-in-amhara-towns/ n.d.; Internal Displacement Monitoring Centre (IDMC) 2023b).

5.5 Challenges in Maintaining ART Adherence

For people living with HIV in conflict-affected settings, maintaining antiretroviral therapy (ART) adherence presents one of the most significant challenges. Frequent displacement due to insecurity makes it difficult for patients to access ART consistently, leading to treatment interruptions, increased viral loads, and the emergence of drug-resistant strains of HIV (Ouma et al. 2021). In many IDP and refugee camps across Africa, stockouts and supply chain failures mean that even when patients are willing to continue treatment, they are unable to do so due to a lack of available medication (Boeyink et al. 2022).

Healthcare infrastructure in conflict zones is often severely compromised, with many trained personnel either fleeing the violence or lacking the necessary resources to continue providing HIV services (Dellie et al. 2024; Amodu et al. 2020). This creates an environment where PLHIV are forced to navigate a fragmented and unreliable healthcare system with little continuity of care. In situations where ART is available, many displaced individuals lack the proper documentation or medical history required to access treatment, leading to discontinuity in their care (Cazabat 2020). The absence of electronic medical records in many African countries further complicates efforts to track and maintain ART adherence among displaced populations (Kodo et al. 2024).

5.6 Stigma and Discrimination in Refugee Camps and Host Communities

HIV-related stigma and discrimination remain significant barriers to treatment and care in displacement settings across Africa. Internally displaced persons and refugees living with HIV often face discrimination from both their host communities and fellow IDPs, creating an environment of fear and isolation (Amodu et al. 2020). Some healthcare facilities in host countries deny HIV-positive IDPs access to essential services due to misconceptions about HIV transmission or limited resources.

Women living with HIV in IDP and refugee camps face a particularly high burden of discrimination. Many are blamed for spreading the virus and subjected to violence or abandonment by their families (Kim et al. 2009). Pregnant women living with HIV are often reluctant to seek maternal health services due to fear of being stigmatized, leading to higher mother-to-child transmission rates (Amodu et al. 2020). Addressing HIV-related stigma requires community-led awareness campaigns, peer-support groups, and legal protections to ensure equitable healthcare access for displaced populations.

5.7 Gender-Based Violence and Sexual Health in Africa's Displaced Populations

Gender-based violence (GBV) is a pervasive issue affecting displaced populations in Africa, exacerbated by armed conflicts, forced migration, and systemic inequalities. In conflict-affected regions, sexual violence has been widely documented as a weapon of war, used to instill fear, exert control, and destabilize communities (Brown 2012; United Nations 2024b). Women and girls bear the brunt of this violence, often suffering profound physical and psychological consequences, with limited access to justice or healthcare services (United Nations 2024b). A cross-sectional study in three internally displaced sites in Northern Ethiopia has estimated the one-year prevalence of GBV to be was 37.9% (Workie et al. 2023).

The use of sexual violence as a weapon of war is a well-documented phenomenon in many African conflicts. In Ethiopia's Amhara and Tigray regions, reports indicate systematic sexual violence against women and girls during conflict, perpetuated by both state and non-state actors (Dellie et al. 2024). Similar patterns have been observed in Northern Uganda, where displaced women, particularly sex workers, experience high levels of client-perpetrated GBV due to socio-economic vulnerabilities and lack of legal protections (Ouma et al. 2021). Survivors of such violence face extreme stigma, often preventing them from seeking medical and legal assistance.

Access to post-rape care and emergency contraception remains inadequate in many displacement settings. Studies show that emergency contraception and post-exposure prophylaxis (PEP) are often unavailable due to resource constraints, weak healthcare infrastructure, and sociocultural taboos surrounding sexual violence. Many survivors delay seeking care due to fear of stigma, inadequate transportation, and a lack of healthcare facilities equipped to handle sexual violence cases. Without timely medical intervention, survivors are at increased risk of unintended pregnancies, sexually transmitted infections (STIs), and long-term reproductive health complications. Strengthening post-rape care services through mobile clinics, rape crisis centres, and better healthcare provider training is essential to improving outcomes for survivors.

The psychological impact of GBV on displaced women is profound. Many survivors suffer from post-traumatic stress disorder (PTSD), depression, and anxiety, yet psychosocial support remains largely inaccessible in many humanitarian settings (Boeyink et al. 2022). Displaced women in Somalia and the Democratic Republic of Congo (DRC) rely heavily on informal social networks, such as faith-based groups and community elders, for emotional support, given the scarcity of formal mental health services (Boeyink et al. 2022). However, these networks may not always provide appropriate trauma-informed care. Community-based interventions, including peer support groups, culturally sensitive counselling, and the integration of psychosocial care into humanitarian programmes, are necessary to address the complex emotional needs of survivors.

The availability and quality of health services for displaced populations vary widely across Africa. A scoping review of IDP women's health in Africa highlights severe gaps in maternal care, contraceptive access, and STI management (Amodu et al. 2020). Many health facilities in conflict zones lack trained personnel, essential medications, and safe environments for women seeking reproductive health services (Boeyink et al. 2022). In some cases, health services are only accessible through humanitarian organizations, further underscoring the need for government investment in healthcare infrastructure.

Humanitarian organizations play a pivotal role in addressing GBV and sexual health disparities among displaced populations. Agencies such as UNHCR, WHO, and Médecins Sans Frontières (MSF) provide emergency medical care, legal aid, and survivor-centred services (Amodu et al. 2020). However, funding constraints, logistical challenges, and political barriers limit the scale and impact of these interventions. Greater investment in long-term development programmes, partnerships with local NGOs, and community-led initiatives is necessary to enhance the sustainability of GBV response efforts (Boeyink et al. 2022).

Integrating sexual health services into primary healthcare systems is a critical step toward addressing the needs of displaced women. Frontline healthcare workers should receive training on GBV screening, trauma-informed care, and medical management of sexual violence cases (Amodu et al. 2020). Expanding mobile clinics and telehealth services can help reach displaced populations in remote areas, while strengthening referral pathways between healthcare providers, legal institutions, and social services can ensure survivors receive comprehensive care (Boeyink et al. 2022). Additionally, developing culturally sensitive outreach programmes can promote awareness of sexual health rights and available services, encouraging more survivors to seek support.

Despite the progress made in addressing GBV, significant challenges remain. Many survivors continue to face stigma, discrimination, and systemic barriers to accessing care and justice. While humanitarian organizations provide essential services, long-term solutions require policy reforms, increased government investment, and the establishment of survivor-centred care models (Amodu et al. 2020). Strengthening the healthcare system's capacity to provide trauma-informed sexual and reproductive healthcare, expanding psychosocial support networks, and improving legal frameworks are crucial steps toward addressing GBV among displaced populations in Africa.

In conclusion, gender-based violence remains a critical public health and human rights issue in African displacement settings. Addressing the intersection of GBV and sexual health requires a coordinated, multi-sectoral approach involving healthcare providers, humanitarian organizations, policymakers, and local communities. Ensuring equitable access to medical, psychological, and legal support for survivors is essential to breaking the cycle of violence and fostering resilience among displaced populations. A sustainable and survivor-centred response will not only improve health outcomes but also contribute to broader efforts in gender equity and human rights protection across the region.

References

Aboagye RG et al (2023) Sexual violence and self-reported sexually transmitted infections among women in sub-Saharan Africa. J Biosoc Sci 55(2):292–305

Adeola R (2021) The protection and assistance of internally displaced persons under the Kampala Convention: an institutional approach. Refugee Surv Q 40(2):173–202

African Union's (Kampala Convention) (2009) African Union convention for the protection and assistance of internally displaced persons in Africa (Kampala Convention). African Union

Amodu OC, Richter MS, Salami BO (2020) A scoping review of the health of conflict-induced internally displaced women in Africa. Int J Environ Res Public Health 17(4):1280

Arage MW et al (2023) Exploring the health consequences of armed conflict: the perspective of Northeast Ethiopia, 2022: a qualitative study. BMC Public Health 23(1):2078

Boeyink C, Ali-Salad MA, Baruti EW et al (2022) Pathways to care: IDPs seeking health support and justice for sexual and gender-based violence through social connections in Garowe and Kismayo, Somalia and South Kivu, DRC. J Migr Health 6:100129

Brown C (2012) Rape as a weapon of war in the Democratic Republic of the Congo. Torture 22(1):24–30

Cazabat C (2020) Women and girls in internal displacement. Internal Displacement Monitoring Centre (IDMC)

Chen MI et al (2008) Reproductive health for refugees by refugees in Guinea II: sexually transmitted infections. Confl Heal 2(14):23
Dafallah A et al (2023) Destruction, disruption and disaster: Sudan's health system amidst armed conflict. Confl Heal 17(1):43
Dellie E, Salelew E, Fetene SM et al (2024) Gender-based violence among women and girls in conflict-affected areas of Northeast Amhara, Ethiopia. Front Glob Women's Health 5:1453149
Desrosiers A et al (2020) A systematic review of sexual and reproductive health interventions for young people in humanitarian and lower-and-middle-income country settings. BMC Public Health 20(1):666
van der Eem L et al (2016) Evaluation of syndromic management guidelines for treatment of sexually transmitted infections in South African women. Trop Med Int Health: TM & IH 21(9):1138–1146
Fahme SA et al (2024) Intersecting social-ecological vulnerabilities to and lived experiences of sexually transmitted infections among Syrian refugee women in Lebanon: a qualitative study. PLOS Glob Public Health 4(8):e0003507
Fiedler C (2023) What do we know about how armed conflict affects social cohesion? a review of the empirical literature. Int Stud Rev 25(3):viad030
World Health Organization (2021) Guidelines for the management of symptomatic sexually transmitted infections. World Health Organization, Geneva. Licence: CC BY-NC-SA 3.0 IGO
Gupta V, Sharma VK (2019) Syndromic management of sexually transmitted infections: a critical appraisal and the road ahead. Natl Med J India 32:147–152
Holt BY et al (2003) Planning STI/HIV prevention among refugees and mobile populations: situation assessment of Sudanese refugees. Disasters 27(1):1–15
https://www.amnesty.org/en/latest/news/2022/02/ethiopia-tigrayan-forces-murder-rape-and-pillage-in-attacks-on-civilians-in amhara-towns/ (n.d.)
Internal Displacement Monitoring Centre (IDMC) (2023a) Conflicts causing record-level of forced displacement in Africa
Internal Displacement Monitoring Centre (IDMC) (2023b) Internal displacement in Africa from 2009 to 2023
International Planned Parenthood Federation (n.d.) Ensuring SRHR in humanitarian crises: what you need to know. International Planned Parenthood Federation. https://www.ippf.org/stories/ensuring-srhr-humanitarian-crises-what-you-need-know. Accessed 6 Mar 2025
Kavulikirwa OK (2024) Intersecting realities: exploring the nexus between armed conflicts in eastern Democratic Republic of the Congo and Global Health. One Health (Amsterdam, Netherlands) 19:100849
Kelly L (2021) Lessons on implementing IDP protection law and policy K4D Helpdesk Report. Institute of Development Studies
Kidie AA et al (2025) A study on sexual violence among women in Northern Ethiopia's 2022 conflict: mixed methods. Front Glob Womens Health 5:1340038
Kim AA, Malele F, Kaiser R, Mama N, Kinkela T, Mantshumba JC, Hynes M, De Jesus S, Musema G, Kayembe PK et al (2009) HIV infection among internally displaced women and women residing in river populations along The Congo River, Democratic Republic of Congo. AIDS Behav 13:914–920
Kodo TK et al (2024) The impact of armed conflict on services and outcomes related to maternal and reproductive health in North Wollo, Amhara, Ethiopia: a qualitative study. Int J Women's Health 16:1055–1066
Kvasnevska Y et al (2024) Impact of war-associated factors on spread of sexually transmitted infections: a systemic review. Front Public Health 12:1366600
Mayaud P et al (1997) STD rapid assessment in Rwandan refugee camps in Tanzania. Genitourin Med 73(1):33–38
Mesfin B et al (2023) The effect of armed conflict on treatment interruption, its outcome and associated factors among chronic disease patients in North East, Amhara, Ethiopia, 2022. Patient Relat Outcome Meas 14:243–251
Moffa MA, Feng X, Mpagazi J et al (2025) Sexually transmitted infections and migration in Uganda: a population-based study. Sex Transm Infect 101(1):27–33. Published 2025 Jan 29
Mohamed EMA, Lucero-Prisno D-E (2025) The effects of Sudan's armed conflict on economy and health: a perspective. Health Sci Rep 8(2):e70424
Morris K (2009) Research vital to improve sexual health of refugees. Lancet Infect Dis 9(4):212
Murphy M et al (2023) Risk and protective factors for violence against women and girls living in conflict and natural disaster-affected settings: a systematic review. Trauma Violence Abuse 24(5):3328
Okorafor KA et al (2024) Exploring sexual and reproductive health needs, barriers, and coping strategies of internally displaced women of reproductive ages in north-Central Nigeria: a qualitative analysis. PLoS One 19(12):e0309317
Otieno FO et al (2014) Evaluation of syndromic management of sexually transmitted infections within the Kisumu Incidence Cohort Study. Int J STD AIDS 25(12):851–859
Ouma S, Ndejjo R, Abbo C et al (2021) Client-perpetrated gender-based violence among female sex workers in conflict-affected Northern Uganda: a cross-sectional study. BMJ Open 11:e046894
Padovese V, Knapp A (2021) Challenges of managing skin diseases in refugees and migrants. Dermatol Clin 39(1):101–115
Siraw A, Addis K, Addis A, Habtetsion M (2019) The prevalence of symptomatic sexually transmitted diseases among refugees in Addis Ababa, Ethiopia. Ethiop J Health Biomed Sci [Internet]. 9(1):15–27. 2019 [cited 2025 Feb 19]
Tewabe DS et al (2024) Gender-based violence in the context of armed conflict in Northern Ethiopia. Confl Heal 18(1):1
Tol WA et al (2013) Sexual and gender-based violence in areas of armed conflict: a systematic review of mental

health and psychosocial support interventions. Confl Heal 7(1):16

Tsadik M et al (2024) Armed conflict and maternal health service utilization in Ethiopia's Tigray region: a community-based survey. BMC Public Health 24(1):2840

United Nations (2024a) Remarks of SRSG Pramila patten at the security council open debate on preventing conflict-related sexual violence through demilitarization and gender-responsive arms control, New York. United Nations. Accessed 6 Mar 2025. https://www.un.org/sexualviolenceinconflict/statement/remarks-of-srsg-pramila-patten-at-the-security-council-open-debate-on-preventing-conflict-related-sexual-violence-through-demilitarization-and-gender-responsive-arms-control-new-yor/

United Nations (2024b). Conflict-related sexual violence: Report of the United Nations Secretary-General (S/2024/292). Office of the Special Representative of the Secretary-General on Sexual Violence in Conflict.

United Nations Office for the Coordination of Humanitarian Affairs (OCHA) (2004) Guiding principles on internal displacement, 2nd edn. United Nations

United Nations Population Fund (2023) "Sometimes She Was Desperate": how survivors of sexual violence in the democratic republic of the Congo are healing with the help of UNFPA's Frontline Workers. UNFPA

Vasylyeva TI et al (2022) Left behind on the path to 90-90-90: understanding and responding to HIV among displaced people. J Int AIDS Soc 25(11):e26031

Vesco P, Baliki G, Brück T, Döring S, Eriksson A, Fjelde H, Guha-Sapir D, Hall J, Knutsen CH, Leis MR et al (2025) The impacts of armed conflict on human development: a review of the literature. World Dev 187:106806

White RG et al (2008) Low effectiveness of syndromic treatment services for curable sexually transmitted infections in rural South Africa. Sex Transm Infect 84(7):528–534

Workie K, Tinsae T, Salelew E et al (2023) Gender-based violence and its associated factors among internally displaced women in Northwest Ethiopia: a cross-sectional study. BMC Women's Health 23:166. https://doi.org/10.1186/s12905-023-02306-2

World Health Organization (2020) Quality of care in fragile, conflict-affected and vulnerable settings: taking action. World Health Organization, Geneva. Licence: CC BY-NC-SA 3.0 IGO

Health Outcomes in Migrant Survivors of Sexual Violence and Abuse

6

Lorna O'Doherty, Grace Carter, and Edward Ong Yung Chet

Contents

Abstract

Sexual violence is common in migration contexts, intersecting with people's motivations for migrating, traversing volatile territories and borders, and circumstances encountered in destination settings. This chapter draws together the research and evidence on the consequences of exposure to sexual and gender-based violence for well-being. It considers how and why access to and experiences of care may differ between survivors of sexual violence who are migrant, refugee, and displaced people and those who are not. In doing so, it informs approaches to recognising risks and needs of migrant people and their families in different health settings and tailoring responses to be more trauma-competent which includes a sensitivity to diverse cultural backgrounds, reducing linguistic barriers and eradicating the potential for secondary traumas in

L. O'Doherty (✉) · G. Carter
Centre for Healthcare and Community Transformation, Coventry University, Coventry, UK
e-mail: lorna.odoherty@coventry.ac.uk; grace.carter@coventry.ac.uk

E. O. Y. Chet
University of Roehampton, London, UK
e-mail: edward.ong@roehampton.ac.uk

V. Padovese, I. Rossoni (eds.), *Intersections of Sexual Health, Migration and Sexualised Violence*, Sustainable Development Goals Series, https://doi.org/10.1007/978-3-032-20707-4_6

the provision of care and support that arise from racial and other forms of discrimination.

Keywords

Gender-based violence · Sexual violence · Migration · Post-migration · Mental health · PTSD · Outcomes · Survivors

6.1 Introduction

> [1]The guards arrived, they were armed, they fired in the air, they wanted to take my daughter, I shouted that they had to kill me if they wanted her. They kept shooting, I was on my knees, hands on my head, I really thought that I will die in this moment
> *A woman from Ivory Coast describes her experience of migrating to France*

Violence against women is a global public health and clinical problem of pandemic proportions (WHO 2021). Violence affects the health and well-being of women and their children, with the global cost of violence against women and girls estimated at approximately 2% of global gross domestic product (UN Women 2016). One in three women across the world has been a victim of intimate partner violence, or sexual violence perpetrated by someone who is not a partner or ex-partner (WHO 2013). Rates for lifetime exposure vary from around 20% to 40% across the major global regions; however, zones with marked economic and political instability and war and conflict are associated with particularly high risk (WHO 2013). According to the WHO (2021), 40% to 50% of women and girls in locations like Afghanistan, Bangladesh, Bolivia, the Democratic Republic of the Congo, South Sudan, and Zambia reported they experienced sexual or domestic violence. Rates are higher again among survivors of human trafficking (WHO 2021): one study of individuals who were in contact with support services in England found that 95% of women trafficked for sexual exploitation, half of women trafficked for domestic servitude, and 20% of women trafficked for labour exploitation reported having been forced to have sex while trafficked (Oram et al. 2016). The ever-changing nature of mobility patterns, regardless of necessity or choice, and shifts in international and domestic policy, law reform, social and economic condition, and service provision/access underscore the need for high-quality evidence upon which to develop and deliver interventions to support migrant survivors and train the professionals and organisations that work with them.

6.1.1 Definitions and Scope

Sexual violence and abuse is a global public health concern and a violation of human rights. It sits within a wider context of gender-based violence. Exposure to sexual violence has serious short- and long-term consequences for a person's health and well-being and for their capacity to participate in education, work, family, and community life. The World Health Organisation (2021, p.7) uses the following definition for sexual violence:

> being forced, coerced or threatened to perform any unwanted sexual act; this could include rape, attempted rape, unwanted sexual touching or non-contact forms of sexual violence.

Sexual violence is distinguished from intimate partner violence which may or may not involve sexual violence and is defined by the WHO (2013, p.9) as 'behaviour by an intimate partner that causes psychological abuse and controlling behaviours. This definition covers violence by both current and former spouses and other intimate partners'. The WHO defines sexual violence that occurs in the context of an intimate relationship as 'being physically forced to have sexual intercourse when you do not want to; having sexual intercourse out of fear for what your partner might do or through coercion; and/or being forced to do something sexual that you

[1]Anonymised quotes from an unpublished study by the lead author are provided throughout to illustrate people's experiences of sexual violence in the context of migration. The research relates to the CAPTIVE Project (Cultural Agent Promoting & Targeting Interventions vs Violence & Enslavement) funded by the European Commission under grant agreement JUST/2015/RDAP/AG/VICT/9243.

consider humiliating or degrading' (WHO 2021, p.6). Sexual violence disproportionately affects women and girls and those with diverse sexual and gender identities. However, it is acknowledged that experience and perpetration of sexual violence transcend all gender, sexuality, social, cultural, and class categories.

Sexual exploitation is closely connected to sexual violence and refers to circumstances where an individual or group takes advantage of an imbalance of power to coerce, control, manipulate, or deceive an individual of any age and exploits them through violence (or the threat of violence), for the financial or other advantage of the perpetrator or facilitator, or in exchange for something the victim needs or wants (Department for Education 2017). The victim may have been exploited even if the activity appeared consensual or did not involve physical contact. Sexual exploitation has particular relevance in the context of migration.

6.1.2 Sexual Violence and Migration

> They arrested us when we walked in peaceful demonstration; they kidnapped and locked us up. When we are locked into prisons, the men rape all the women, sometimes it is ten men who pass, they rape us in front of the other women *A woman from the Democratic Republic of the Congo explains about her experience before leaving for Europe*

Sexual violence, intimate partner violence, family/domestic violence, and the broader category of gender-based violence and abuse are implicated in the reasons people migrate, especially for women and girls and people from gender and sexual minorities. People may choose to leave their country of origin in search of environments that promote greater gender equality and associated economic opportunity and safety, including reducing risks of sexual violence, intimate partner violence, domestic/family violence, and other forms of gender-based violence and abuse for themselves, their families, and communities (Cummings et al. 2015). People may leave their homes to flee persecution or human rights violations such as torture and sexual violence. It is known that the incidence of sexual violence increases during times of war and conflict (De Schrijver et al. 2018; Freedman 2010; United Nations 2024). Taken together, there is evidence of sexual and gender-based violence and abuse as acute or cumulative 'push' factors for migration (WHO 2022).

> Selling people is normal in Libya *A Nigerian woman interviewed in Italy*

Risk of exposure to abuse and exploitation, including sexual forms of abuse and exploitation, is aggravated over the course of a person's migration journey and interacts with individuals' reasons for migration, cultural and ethnic identities, routes taken, duration of journeys, and access to resources (WRC 2016). A particularly concerning issue is the migration and involuntary displacement of children and young people—overcrowded refugee camps are common and are unsafe and create risks for sexual violence and exploitation of children and young people (Kwankye et al. 2021). Recent studies (see Andersson Nystedt et al. 2024) also suggest that young migrants in Europe, especially those from conflict zones, are particularly vulnerable to sexual violence during their transit. However, the very limited research into exposure to sexual violence in this sub-population means the problem is under-recognised which in turn perpetuates a continued lack of attention to the issue and lack of evidence for informing interventions, identifying victims and survivors, and facilitating access to care (Digidiki and Bhabha 2018; Jud et al. 2020). Immigration may be the most politicised issue of our time. For example, Europe and its leaders scramble to deliver measures to stem the flow of people. However, in practice these measures may undermine human rights and aggravate a host of risks for migrants which includes sexual violence against women and girls.

> I didn't even know what my rights were, and what I can do here; my husband used to say 'I can send you back, you're in my control, the law in this country [is such that] when husband calls a wife here, he can do anything to her and she has no rights' *A Pakistani woman describes experience of arranged marriage to a man in the United Kingdom*

Exposure to sexual violence and abuse is also an appalling reality for many people at the end of their journey and in post-migration environments. Risk of abuse in destination locations can interact with age, socio-economic status, trauma and health status, education, skills and capacity to work, linguistic capabilities, immigration status, and whether people are held in detention settings or not (Şenses 2020). International students are an important migrant subgroup to consider, with millions of students/young people travelling internationally to attend universities each year. Sexual violence is particularly prevalent in university populations (Black et al. 2011), prompted by a high-risk context of increasing independence and risk behaviours, with estimates suggesting 25% (5–10% exposed to rape) of female students and 5% of male students experience sexual assault (Rosenberg et al. 2019; Fedina et al. 2018). Several studies have also highlighted the high prevalence of intimate partner abuse and reproductive coercion in this population (Grace et al. 2022). International students may be more at risk of sexual violence than domestic students (Brubaker et al. 2017) and/or may experience greater difficulties accessing healthcare and emotional support. For example, asking for help may be impossible if the young person comes from a culture where talking about sex and relationships is taboo (O'Doherty et al. 2024) or the person is experiencing social isolation.

A study of refugees from six conflict countries about their exposure to violence concluded that gender-based abuse persists across the span of the refugee experience, but that there is a shift in the perpetrators and types of abuse experienced (Wirtz et al. 2013). For example, opportunistic violence, often manifested by rape, occurred during transit when women depended on others to reach their destination. Domestic abuse was more common in the post-migration environment/host. Overall, individuals' access to safe housing, health services and other personal, family and community resources; the legal and social protections afforded to migrants (including those on student visas) and refugee people; and the prevailing socio-political context and public attitudes to immigration all play a role in risks and the responses survivors receive if or when they seek help in the aftermath of exposure to sexual and gender-based violence (Pertek et al. 2021; Phillimore et al. 2022).

> 'We, the housekeepers, don't have any rights. Because if I don't work, I won't renew my documents and the pressure... you know? The pressure is the first thing. A woman puts up with many things. I was raped at my job and I didn't tell. For surviving, I've borne what nobody can bear' *A Moroccan woman living in Spain highlights the subjugation of migrant women*

There is significant potential for a wide range of trauma in the lives and histories of refugee, asylum-seeking and migrant people, which could include recent or non-recent exposure to sexual violence along with experiences of displacement, bereavement and loss, racism, other forms of discrimination, exploitation, and social and economic disadvantage. Therefore, it is essential to promote and implement trauma-informed first principles across public services and in the provision of healthcare. This requires attending to the circumstances of people's lives and the barriers they face in communicating which arise from their past experiences of interacting with public and government agencies and authorities in countries of origin or post-migration.

6.2 Mental Health Experiences and Health Outcomes

In acknowledging the overlap between migration, sexual violence, and mental health (Fig. 6.1), we start this section with an overview of how

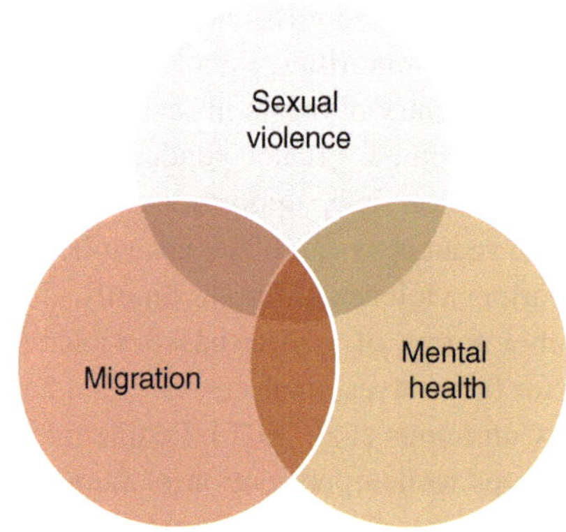

Fig. 6.1 Overlap in key themes of the chapter

mental health outcomes interact with migration experiences. We subsequently examine the evidence for mental health consequences common to any population, group or individual affected by sexual violence and then also attend to the particular risks, problems and experiences of survivors who also have migration experience.

6.2.1 Migration and Mental Health

> I couldn't sleep because in my country there was a lot of violence. I thought 'these men are going to rape us during the night...' and I kept protecting my little daughter with a knife I stole from a bar *A woman from Mexico describes trying to sleep at night after migrating to Spain*

Migration is a universal and a historical phenomenon that is typically driven by a variety of factors, including economic needs, the quest for better living conditions, escape from conflict, and environmental changes. However, migration also has an intricate relationship with mental health, which is underscored by complexities and a variety of challenges migrants face and how these impact their psychological wellbeing throughout different stages of their immigration (Virupaksha et al. 2014). This increased risk can be attributed to various factors encountered during different stages of migration: before departure, during transit, and after arrival (Jannesari et al. 2020). For instance, the pre-migration phase often involves difficult decisions and may be accompanied by fear and uncertainty. The transit phase can expose individuals to harsh conditions, trauma, and exploitation, which can lead to acute stress reactions. The post-migration phase brings challenges such as cultural adjustment, language barriers, loneliness and isolation, discrimination, and the pressure to assimilate, which can influence mental health literacy and individuals' willingness to seek care, which may further contribute to chronic stress and mental health disorders like depression, anxiety, and post-traumatic stress disorder (PTSD; Jannesari et al. 2020; Virupaksha et al. 2014).

Further evidence also indicates that post-migration factors are particularly poignant, as they may mediate the impact of pre-migration stressors (Khawaja et al. 2008; Miller and Rasmussen 2010; Watters 2001). For example, research indicates that asylum seekers are more likely to develop mental health problems compared to both refugees and native populations (Ryan et al. 2009). These mental health problems are also often exacerbated by poor living conditions and prolonged detention, the lack of social support and experiences of social isolation, unemployment and financial instability, legal and residency uncertainty, as well as experiences of discrimination and social exclusion (Jannesari et al. 2020). Furthermore, the stigma associated with mental health issues may be heightened in some cultural groups (Leamy et al. 2011) and play a role in migrant people delaying/avoiding help-seeking and the deterioration of health (Javed et al. 2021).

6.2.2 Sexual Violence and Mental Health

In making sense of the impacts of exposure to sexual violence on health for migrant people, we firstly examine common responses to sexual trauma. A robust body of evidence links exposure to sexual violence to poor mental health experiences and outcomes in a range of populations, including community (MacMillan et al. 2001), young people (Bentivegna and Patalay 2022; Khadr et al. 2018), men (Easton and Kong 2017), migrant women (Hossain et al. 2010), individuals affected by substance misuse (Austin and Short 2020), survivors of domestic abuse (Tarzia et al. 2018), victims of human trafficking (Altun et al. 2017; Ottisova et al. 2016) and those accessing mental health care (Hughes et al. 2019; Khalifeh et al. 2015; Oram et al. 2017) and forensic health services (O'Doherty et al. 2024). The gender gap observed in the prevalence of common mental illnesses, including PTSD and specific PTSD symptoms (Guina et al. 2019), may be down to women and girls' increased exposure to sexual violence and abuse.

Outcomes examined in studies of the mental health consequences of abuse are wide-ranging and include distress, self-harm, suicidality, anxiety, depression, substance misuse, prescription drug use, and PTSD (Khalifeh et al. 2015; Oram 2019; O'Doherty et al. 2023; 2024). Studies also highlight the impacts on social impairment, emotional dysregulation (Villalta et al. 2020), sleep problems such as increased nightmare-related distress, sleep paralysis, and restless sleep (Steine et al. 2012) and dissociation (Brokke et al. 2022). Generally, people affected by mental health problems carry a much greater risk of sexual violence victimisation than those without mental health problems, with research suggesting a sixfold higher odds of recent/past year sexual victimisation among those with severe mental health issues compared with the general population (Khalifeh et al. 2016). Further, as with domestic abuse, the relationship between sexual violence and poor mental health may be bidirectional, where exposure to abuse leads to poor mental health, and having mental health difficulties places a person at increased risk of victimisation (O'Doherty et al. 2024; Oram et al. 2017). There are also serious implications for trying to parent and raise children when managing the psychological impacts of sexual violence and other traumas associated with migration, suggestive of intergenerational trauma.

> 'My daughter, she is very quiet, she doesn't laugh, she doesn't know happiness' *A woman from the Democratic Republic of the Congo talks about the long term impacts of her own trauma on her daughter's life and mental wellbeing (in the UK)*

6.2.3 Sexual Violence and PTSD

PTSD is a common and debilitating consequence of exposure to a traumatic incident or series of incidents. It is the most frequently investigated effect of exposure to rape, sexual assault and abuse, both in terms of understanding the mental health sequelae (Liu et al. 2017) and for evaluating interventions aiming to alleviate the mental health effects of sexual trauma (O'Doherty et al. 2023). PTSD can develop in response to a disturbing, frightening, or dangerous event or experience. Based on the Diagnostic and Statistical Manual (DSM)-5, PTSD involves four symptom domains: (1) re-experiencing symptoms, such as flashbacks and nightmares; (2) avoidance, such as staying away from places, events, or objects that are reminders of the experience; (3) arousal and reactivity symptoms, such as difficulties with concentration and sleep; and (4) mood and cognition problems, such as difficulties recalling details of the traumatic experience and feelings of social isolation (American Psychiatric Association 2013). The sympathetic nervous system response triggered during an extremely threatening experience or event such as rape or sexual assault to promote survival at the time comes at the expense of crippling, long-term nervous system hyperactivity and the exaggerated responsiveness characteristic of PTSD. PTSD has been described as a Trauma Spectrum Disorder (Bremner 2002), associated with a specific neurobiological profile and with clear links to stress. Within the DSM-5, PTSD sits in the category of Trauma- and Stressor-related Disorders (American Psychiatric Association 2013). Included in this category is Acute Stress Disorder, a DSM-5 diagnosis that applies in the first month after a traumatic event and understood as a precursor to PTSD in some cases.

The World Health Organisation World Mental Health Surveys gathered data about mental health in 24 countries ($n = 68{,}894$) (Kessler et al. 2017) and provide some important insights into PTSD among survivors of sexual violence and abuse. Firstly, across 29 traumatic experiences (or events) measured, the trauma types with the highest proportions of PTSD burden identified worldwide were rape (13.1%) and other forms of sexual assault (15.1%). Secondly, this research examined the conditional risk for PTSD after trauma; it reported that one in five people exposed to rape and over 1 in 10 of those with other forms of sexual assault developed PTSD relative to 4% across the 29 traumas assessed. A further relevant finding from the Mental Health Surveys concerns the persistence of PTSD. Time to recovery, defined as the number of months until respondents stopped having any PTSD symptoms, was 110 months (9 years) for survivors of any intimate partner-perpetrated or sexual violence and abuse. This and other research (O'Doherty et al. 2024) note that a history of prior trauma, and in particular physical or sexual violence, increases a person's vulnerability to future PTSD across the full range of trauma types (Liu et al. 2017; Kessler et al. 2018). This finding has relevance to asylum-seeking, refugee and migrant people generally, who are at risk of multiple traumatic exposures (e.g., war-related trauma, accidents, and natural disasters, witnessing death or injury).

6.3 Access to Care After Exposure to Sexual Violence for Migrant and Other Groups

In the aftermath of exposure to sexual violence, victims and survivors may present for care and support for their emotional, sexual, and physical well-being and to secure their safety and rights to justice through a range of agencies and systems. These include policing/law enforcement, a range of health settings, social and child protection services, education, sexual assault and abuse services, and domestic abuse services as well as other voluntary and community organisations. How a person goes about accessing the care and support they need will be influenced by a complex web of individual, criminogenic, social, economic, and cultural factors. One critical factor for outcomes after sexual violence is the type of support accessed and when it is accessed (i.e. the length of time that has passed since the rape, sexual assault or abuse occurred). Whilst immediate access to evidence-based care is likely to promote better outcomes for survivors, only a small proportion of people access care that is timely. Timeliness is often applied in the context of gathering forensic evidence after sexual assault or rape on the basis that acting quickly gives the greatest chance of securing forensic evidence which may be useful in a criminal case. In the UK, the Faculty of Forensic & Legal Medicine recommends a window of up to 7 days for most sample types, and forensic services are mostly accessible at sexual assault referral centres (SARCs). Yet, of the near one million people sexually victimised (including attempts) in England and Wales each year, half of whom experience the most serious sexual offence of rape, less than 30,000 reach SARCs. One study of people attending SARCs in England reported that 45% of participants accessed a SARC within the 'forensic window' (approximately 7–10 days post-assault) and 38% of the sample underwent a forensic medical examination. There is a strong association between reporting to the police and accessing a SARC/obtaining a forensic medical examination. Thus, with the universal barriers of stigma and shame, together with the difficulties survivors experience in relation to going to the police and/or disclosing soon after sexual violence, there are many factors working against timely medico-legal care. Delayed access to medical care for injuries and access to clinical interventions for preventing pregnancy, HIV and other sexually transmitted infections all have serious and long-term implications for health and wellbeing. It may also mean that survivors miss out on emotional health first aid and referral on to mental health care and specialist providers of post-sexual assault care in the NGO sector.

'Timely' care and support hold various meanings for different contexts, and the importance of survivors perceiving choice in relation to care is acknowledged, including survivors choosing if they would disclose the abuse and when is the best time to ask for or accept help. The stigma associated with sexual violence and the shame commonly experienced by survivors, especially if the crime has been committed by someone known to them, the fear of taking action and the fear of not being believed or worse, being held responsible, are powerful deterrents to seeking help and support. Such barriers exist across nations and cultures but may be heightened in communities that are socially, culturally isolated, or economically deprived. Nellums et al. (2018) have found that healthcare access for people seeking asylum was inhibited by the lack of translators or the use of inappropriate translators (friends and family or male interpreters for women's sexual health services). Many people will actively seek out help for themselves without necessarily disclosing what has happened to them. This could be in primary care, mental health services, sexual health, perinatal care and so on. Ideally these environments should be prepared for all scenarios—survivors requiring care but not wishing to disclose their status as a survivor as well as those for whom disclosure under the right conditions is desirable.

> I went to the GP when my difficulties started. He said 'Why are you wasting your time and my time? You are fine, [there's] nothing wrong with you.' I collapsed so many times at home. I wanted to know what was going on. I knew it was stress, but there is the GP which I can't go to and I can't go straight to hospital. He was Indian, Asian, they do this with their people mostly; if I was English person, he would have treated me better. Now my doctor is an English lady—she referred me to hospital
> *An Indian woman now based in the United Kingdom*

Taking an intersectional approach to analysing access and barriers to care in post-migration environments brings into focus the compounding effects of racialised and other marginalised identities (Crenshaw 1989). Migrant women in Europe face multilayered vulnerabilities, in particular, those associated with the interaction of gender, ethnicity, poverty and immigration status. They are not only at risk of being 'othered' (Grillo 2013) in the receiving country context; they are also at risk of being 'othered' within their own cultural contexts if they reject or attempt to escape subordination and abuse increasing social exclusion and risking psychological and physical harm e.g. forms of 'honour' violence. A lack of language or ethnic diversity in services/at the point of access, prior experiences of racial discrimination in healthcare or coming from a cultural background that denies women equivalent status to men are powerful deterrents to care. The impacts of abuse itself, pressures from family and community and fears about retribution are all part of the complex picture of barriers to escaping abuse or gaining access to the care needed for healing.

There is a large body of evidence that highlights the delayed healthcare seeking by migrant populations (Jannesari et al. 2020; Mohammadifirouzeh et al. 2023; Nellums et al. 2018). This is seen among those in exploitative situations, among people with insecure immigration status and those who are experiencing multiple forms of abuse and control, for example domestic violence and servitude (Allen-Leap et al. 2023) and among those affected by substance misuse (McCann et al. 2016). Intersectionality is a vital tool for (re)designing services to tackle inequities in access to care (generally) for marginalised individuals and those made vulnerable through their migration experiences and status in host countries. Such measures are also pivotal for enabling migrant women and others affected by sexual violence to consider seeking help. One example would be to ensure that campaigns to raise awareness of the options for assistance if a person is a victim of sexual violence are implemented for multiple communities and languages. This means working with grassroots organisations and advocacy agencies with embedded relevant cultural knowledge and experience to develop messages about the unacceptability of violence, highlight consequences for one's own health and wellbeing and that of families, and ways to access help. Such organisations can also work with those onward services to ensure they too are ready to practise with trauma competence and cultural humility (Fig. 6.2).

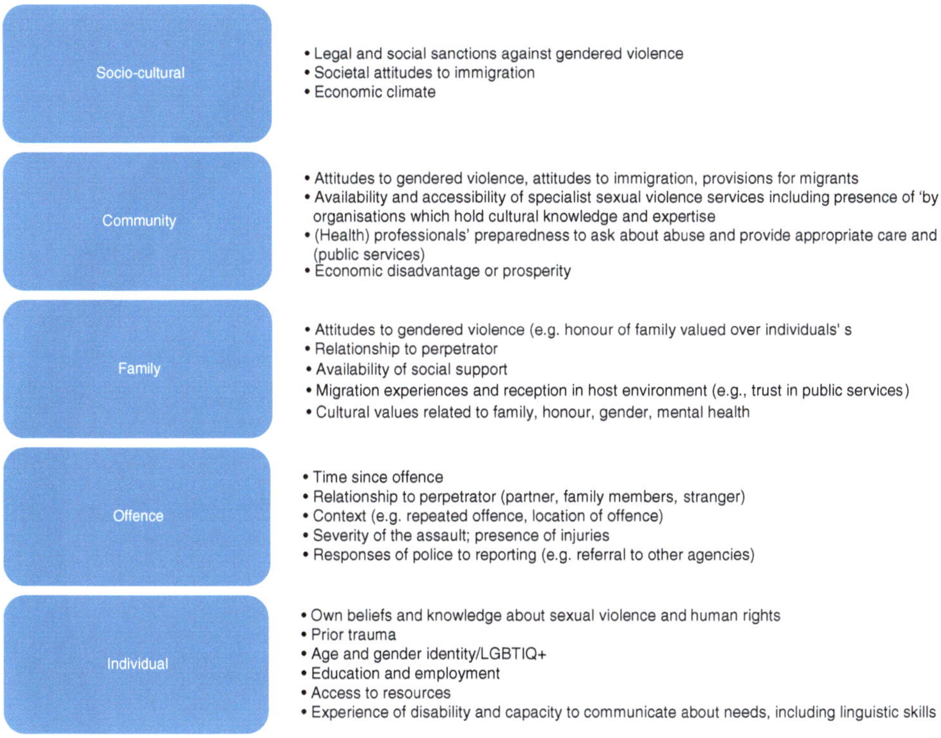

Fig. 6.2 Factors affecting access to care and support among migrant survivors of sexual violence and abuse

6.4 Meeting the Needs of Survivors from Migrant Populations Within Services

We have considered survivors' access needs and how barriers to care and support are particularly extensive for survivors of abuse from migrant backgrounds. Health needs themselves may also be particularly complex for survivors who are migrants. Healthcare environments already struggle to adequately meet the needs of survivors of sexual violence and abuse (O'Doherty et al. 2024). Particular advances in practices, systems and workforce preparedness are required to meet health needs where migration and sexual violence exposure overlap.

Healthcare providers frequently, and often without realising it, encounter survivors of sexual and domestic violence. There is global consensus that healthcare professionals in any health service should know how to identify service users experiencing abuse and respond appropriately to disclosure. This includes demonstrating empathy and offering a non-judgemental response, ensuring confidentiality, and promoting safety and referral to other agencies/services relative to the person's needs, as well as comprehensive care for rape and sexual assault (Fig. 6.3). However, this also means not pressuring a person to disclose and recognising the value in providing accessible information about abuse, its impacts and where to get help and arranging follow-up. Increasingly, it is recognised that addressing violence against women and girls requires a whole-system response (Hegarty et al. 2020). This means supporting and enabling the healthcare professionals undertaking this challenging and sensitive work and recognising professionals may themselves be survivors of abuse (Oram et al. 2017). Whilst clinical settings are widely acknowledged as a suitable setting in which to identify and support victims and survivors of sexual violence (WHO 2013), such environments are not always experienced as places of trust, particularly among mar-

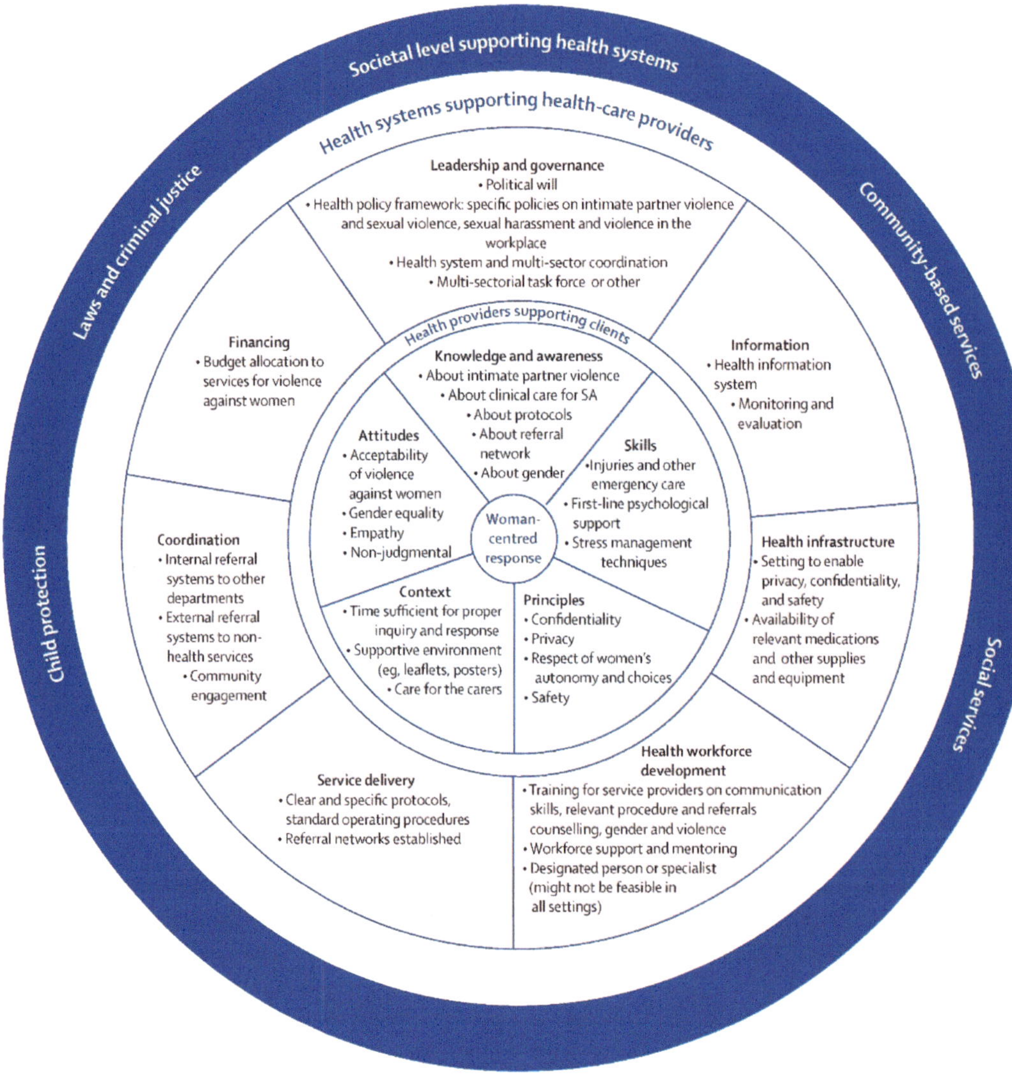

Fig. 6.3 Elements of the health system and healthcare response necessary to address violence against women and girls, including those from migrant backgrounds. (This figure has been adapted from the original article (Colombini et al. 2012) and the previously adapted figure by (García-Moreno et al. 2015). The original article is an open access article distributed under the terms of the Creative Commons Attribution License (http://creativecommons.org/licenses/by/2.0), which permits unrestricted use, distribution, and reproduction in any medium). SA sexual assault

ginalised individuals such as those from migrant, refugee, and asylum-seeking populations.

A consequence of delayed access to care common among survivors from marginalised and migrant backgrounds is many individuals are in crisis by the time they reach services. Further, high rates of untreated mental health disorders are extremely common in migrant populations, and suicidality is often a trigger for healthcare access and response. Such understanding about the nature of vulnerability to PTSD in this population is important for a range of professionals, services, and settings and in targeting support interventions for migrant people, including those accessing care and support for mental health, in the aftermath of sexual violence and other traumas.

When I was in London too, I hadn't heard of these organisations. The environment in which we grew up, I didn't know I had to go to someone to ask for help, but I was suffering within myself. I was admitted to hospital; then, a few organisations came to see me, used to come to my home. They used to give me tablets - every day, then alternate days, and then weekly. Then I found [specialist (migrant) women's service]. *A woman from India who moved to the United Kingdom*

A person's first encounter with care for the consequences of sexual violence may take place in urgent care settings, for example, emergency departments or community mental health teams, underscoring the need for trauma-informed and culturally competent practices in these healthcare environments. Evidence on the prevalence of sexual violence in mental healthcare-seeking populations and consequences for mental health are compelling (Khalifeh et al. 2016). Mental healthcare providers are an important professional group in the context of a health response to sexual and domestic abuse, but these services often overlook the relevance of sexual violence in providing care (O'Doherty et al. 2024).

Clinical guidelines (NICE 2016; WHO 2013) recommend mental health providers routinely enquire about exposure to abuse and enable disclosure as part of clinical assessments, provide support and ensure safety, and treat or refer physical and mental health problems in the context of any sexual or domestic violence. As with other parts of the health system, mental health services need to ensure conditions are appropriate for providers to safely address issues related to violence against women (Fig. 6.3). Evidence from qualitative studies suggests survivors are open to and value being asked about their prior experiences of sexual violence, provided this is done in a judicious and sensitive way. However, there is also considerable evidence of harmful attitudes and behaviours, for example, expressing a cavalier attitude to disclosure of past abuse or questioning survivors in ways that hold them accountable for the abuse they suffered (Fig. 6.4). Contrasting with this, survivors feel empowered in mental health care settings when they can choose to talk about the abuse or not (Fig. 6.5).

Asking about exposure to sexual violence and related forms of gender-based abuse like female genital mutilation (FGM), exploitation and domestic abuse needs to be carried out safely and in a private setting. Health professionals should ensure women have opportunities to be seen without partners, family members, or acquaintances present. Good practices around the enquiry will minimise risks that might arise from a perpetrator or family member being made aware of disclosure, feelings of disempowerment for the survivor, and re-traumatisation. Access to interpreter services is vital and can enhance the flow and understanding of essential information between the parties. A professional service is preferable to using friends and family members. Though barriers like stigma and shame may still be activated where the interpreter shares cultural characteristics with the survivor and thus, this

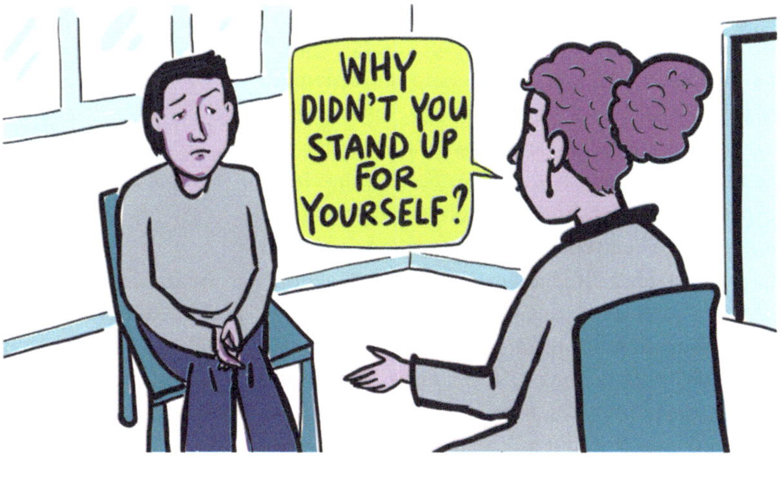

Fig. 6.4 Survivors of sexual violence may encounter blaming attitudes in mental health services. (*Illustration courtesy of Federica Ciotti, in collaboration with MESARCH Multi-study Evaluation of Sexual Assault Referral Centres*)

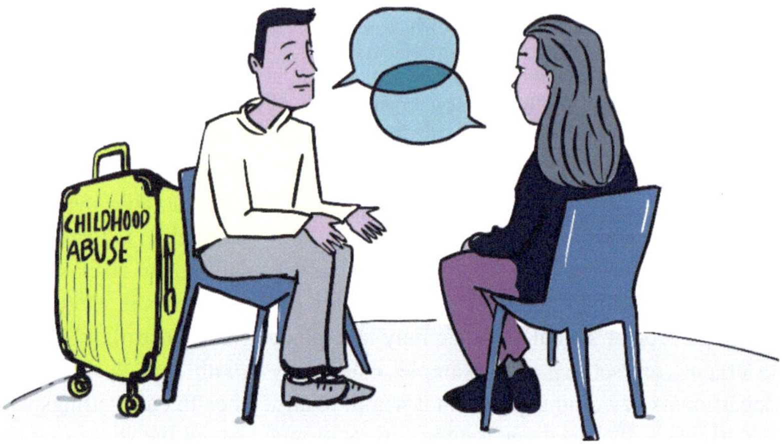

Fig. 6.5 Survivors value being in control of the disclosure process. (*Illustration courtesy of Federica Ciotti, in collaboration with MESARCH Multi-study Evaluation of Sexual Assault Referral Centres)*

can be mitigated through operating to the highest standards of confidentiality and ensuring staff are trauma-informed and culturally aware. Clinicians must respond sensitively, compassionately, and non-judgmentally to disclosure; reassure survivors that they are believed and not to blame for their experiences; and offer information and practical support that responds to concerns and respects the person's autonomy.

> The police did not help at all, they were his friends and males. They made fun of me, being a women and a foreigner – after the police report, I went back to him. The female police officer was very helpful though *A woman from the Philippines now located in Malta*

Beyond ensuring access to health services and mental health support, societies must work to ensure equitable access to justice. Access to justice for sexual violence is a pervasive problem in all parts of the world and demands a global, unified stance towards ensuring perpetrators of sexual violence and abuse are held to account. Marginalised migrant survivors of sexual offences can experience extensive difficulties in accessing justice for all the same reasons they experience barriers to other public services. For crimes that occurred before they arrived, individuals may stand little chance of seeing action against perpetrators. Such injustices have significant implications for health and wellbeing. NGOs like rape crisis centres in the United Kingdom, and especially voluntary organisations that are led or run 'for and by' members of the communities they serve, are a vital part of the landscape for supporting migrant and/or racialised survivors and communities. In addition to a range of interventions and services to tackle isolation and disadvantage, they may support legal action for survivors, such as reporting to the police, and liaise with justice agencies on behalf of the person. They can promote wellness in the context of sexual violence through short-term and long-term counselling and peer support. These organisations also have potential to provide essential advocacy related to housing, employment, education, and health services.

6.5 Implications and Conclusion

> Since I knew Maria, my life changed because I was feeling like I am going to die, I was almost dead because my husband did so many things to me and when I cannot get help, whom to tell about my problems. Yeah but since I knew Maria I was crying, crying, feeling very down, but she used to encourage me. Then I get my life back. I was almost dead. When I used to walk I used to feel the wind would blow and I would fall down *A Ugandan woman shares about her counsellor in the United Kingdom*

Sexual violence is an international public health emergency, which flourishes with global instability, conflict, economic insecurity, and humanitarian crises. The nature of vulnerability shifts as people enter new geographical, social, and cultural spaces and 'become migrants' and immigrants. This is reflected in evidence about migration journeys and the challenges that wait in destination countries. The effects of exposure to sexual violence are widespread, affecting all aspects of a person's health and functioning and severely disrupting a person's capacity to work, engage in their communities and care for their children. Sexual violence (rape and sexual assault) is the leading contributor to the burden of trauma across the globe. The location of migrant women at the intersection of race, immigration and gender makes the actual experience of sexual violence and abuse and seeking assistance qualitatively different from that of individuals in their native setting. Migrant (and often racialised) women suffer from the effects of multiple subordination and polyvictimisation. When these experiences are coupled with institutional expectations from police, immigration agencies, health, housing, and other public services derived from inappropriate, non-intersectional contexts, opportunities for meaningful and timely intervention are greatly limited.

There is an urgent need to increase understanding and awareness of frontline professionals and service providers about the dynamics of structural intersectionality and exercise this understanding in working with migrants and migrant women across sectors. Services need to have specialist reach, including staff that share language and cultural backgrounds; capability around responding to disclosure and handling referral safely and sensitively; cultural competence and confidence to challenge harmful community norms; access to trained interpreters; options for migrant/women to exercise choice (e.g. can request female interviewer for police or immigration interviews); and trauma-informed practice across contexts in which migrant people/women present (Sweeney et al. 2016). There is also a need to maximise the reach of messages to newly arrived and current migrants. This could include ensuring access to information on risks, rights, and services via multiple avenues, including immigration and border control agencies; community groups; and health, public services and other agencies that have contact with migrants and migrant women. Early intervention and long-term engagement with survivors and those at risk are crucial.

Only in bringing these threads to policies, practice and research work with migrant and refugee survivors can we begin to address the toxic and perpetuating mix of marginalisation and violence in the lives of so many.

References

Allen-Leap M, Hooker L, Wild K, Wilson IM, Pokharel B, Taft A (2023) Seeking help from primary healthcare providers in high-income countries: a scoping review of the experiences of migrant and refugee survivors of domestic violence. Trauma Violence Abuse 24(5):3715–3731

Altun S, Abas M, Zimmerman C, Howard LM, Oram S (2017) Mental health and human trafficking: responding to survivors' needs. BJPsych Int 14(1):21–23

American Psychiatric Association (2013) The diagnostic and statistical manual of mental disorders, fifth edition (DSM-5), 5th edn. American Psychiatric Association, Washington, DC. [Google Scholar]

Andersson Nystedt T, Herder T, Agardh A, Asamoah BO (2024) No evidence, no problem? A critical interpretive synthesis of the vulnerabilities to and experiences of sexual violence among young migrants in Europe. Glob Health Action 17(1):2340114

Austin AE, Short NA (2020) Sexual violence, mental health, and prescription opioid use and misuse. Am J Prev Med 59(6):818–827. https://doi.org/10.1016/j.amepre.2020.06.019

Bentivegna F, Patalay P (2022) The impact of sexual violence in mid-adolescence on mental health: a UK population-based longitudinal study. Lancet Psychiatry 9(11):874–883. https://doi.org/10.1016/S2215-0366(22)00271-1

Black MC, Basile KC, Breiding MJ, Smith SG, Walters ML, Merrick MT, Chen J, Stevens MR (2011) The National Intimate Partner and sexual violence survey (NISVS): 2010 summary report. National Center for Injury Prevention and Control, Centers for Disease Control and Prevention, Atlanta, GA

Bremner JD (2002) Does stress damage the brain? Understanding trauma-related disorders from a mind-body perspective. W.W. Norton, New York

Brokke SS, Bertelsen TB, Landrø NI, Haaland VØ (2022) The effect of sexual abuse and dissociation on suicide attempt. BMC Psychiatry 22:1–8

Brubaker SJ, Keegan B, Guadalupe-Diaz XL, Beasley BA (2017) Measuring and reporting campus sexual assault: privilege and exclusion in what we know and what we do. Sociol Compass 11(12):e12543. https://doi.org/10.1111/soc4.12543

Colombini M, Mayhew SH, Ali SH, Shuib R, Watts C (2012) An integrated health sector response to vio-

lence against women in Malaysia: lessons for supporting scale up. BMC Public Health 12:1–10
Crenshaw K (1989) Demarginalizing the intersection of race and sex: a black feminist critique of antidiscrimination doctrine, feminist theory and antiracist politics. Univ Chic Leg Forum 1989, 1(8). Retrieved from: https://chicagounbound.uchicago.edu/uclf/vol1989/iss1/8/?utm_source=chicagounbound.uchicago.edu%2Fuclf%2Fvol1989%2Fiss1%2F8&utm_medium=PDF&utm_campaign=PDFCoverPages
Cummings C, Pacitto J, Lauro D, Foresti M (2015) Why people move: understanding the drivers and trends of migration to Europe. Working Paper 430. Retrieved from: understanding-drivers-migration-Europe.pdf (publishing.service.gov.uk)
Department for Education (2017) Child sexual exploitation Definition and a guide for practitioners, local leaders and decision makers working to protect children from child sexual exploitation. Retrieved from: https://assets.publishing.service.gov.uk/media/5a7f8e3640f0b62305b87dbc/CSE_Guidance_Core_Document_13.02.2017.pdf
De Schrijver L, Vander Beken T, Krahé B, Keygnaert I (2018) Prevalence of sexual violence in migrants, applicants for international protection, and refugees in Europe: a critical interpretive synthesis of the evidence. Int J Environ Res Public Health 15(9):1979
Digidiki V, Bhabha J (2018) Sexual abuse and exploitation of unaccompanied migrant children in Greece: identifying risk factors and gaps in services during the European migration crisis. Child Youth Serv Rev 92:114–121
Easton SD, Kong J (2017) Mental health indicators fifty years later: a population-based study of men with histories of child sexual abuse. Child Abuse Negl 63:273–283
Fedina L, Holmes JL, Backes BL (2018) Campus sexual assault: a systematic review of prevalence research from 2000 to 2015. Trauma Violence Abuse 19(1):76–93
Freedman J (2010) Mainstreaming gender in refugee protection. Camb Rev Int Aff 23(4):589–607. https://doi.org/10.1080/09557571.2010.523820
García-Moreno C, Hegarty K, d'Oliveira AF, Koziol-McLain J, Colombini M, Feder G (2015) The health-systems response to violence against women. Lancet 18;385(9977):1567–79. https://doi.org/10.1016/S0140-6736(14)61837-7. Epub 2014 Nov 21. Erratum in: Lancet. 2015 Apr 18;385(9977):1510. https://doi.org/10.1016/S0140-6736(15)60754-1. PMID: 25467583
Grace KT, Perrin NA, Clough A, Miller E, Glass NE (2022) Correlates of reproductive coercion among college women in abusive relationships: baseline data from the college safety study. J Am Coll Heal 70(4):1204–1211
Grillo R (2013) An excess of alterity? Debating difference in a multicultural society. In: Vertovec S (ed) Anthropology of migration and multiculturalism. Abingdon, Routledge
Guina J, Nahhas RW, Kawalec K, Farnsworth S (2019) Are gender differences in DSM-5 PTSD symptomatology explained by sexual trauma? J Interpers Violence 34(21–22):4713–4740
Hegarty K, McKibbin G, Hameed M, Koziol-McLain J, Feder G, Tarzia L, Hooker L (2020) Health practitioners' readiness to address domestic violence and abuse: a qualitative meta-synthesis. PLoS One 15(6):e0234067
Hossain M, Zimmerman C, Abas M, Light M, Watts C (2010) The relationship of trauma to mental disorders among trafficked and sexually exploited girls and women. Am J Public Health 100(12):2442–2449
Hughes E, Lucock M, Brooker C (2019) Sexual violence and mental health services: a call to action. Epidemiol Psychiatr Sci 28(6):594–597
Jannesari S, Hatch S, Prina M, Oram S (2020) Post-migration social–environmental factors associated with mental health problems among asylum seekers: a systematic review. J Immigr Minor Health 22(5):1055–1064. https://doi.org/10.1007/s10903-020-01025-2
Javed A, Lee C, Zakaria H, Buenaventura RD, Cetkovich-Bakmas M, Duailibi K et al (2021) Reducing the stigma of mental health disorders with a focus on low-and middle-income countries. Asian J Psychiatr 58:102601
Jud A, Pfeiffer E, Jarczok M (2020) Epidemiology of violence against children in migration: a systematic literature review. Child Abuse Negl 108:104634. https://doi.org/10.1016/j.chiabu.2020.104634
Kessler RC, Aguilar-Gaxiola S, Alonso J, Benjet C, Bromet EJ, Cardoso G et al (2017) Trauma and PTSD in the WHO world mental health surveys. Eur J Psychotraumatol 8(sup5):1353383
Kessler RC, Aguilar-Gaxiola S, Alonso J, Bromet EJ, Gureje O, Karam EG et al (2018) The associations of earlier trauma exposures and history of mental disorders with PTSD after subsequent traumas. Mol Psychiatry 23(9):1892–1899
Khalifeh H, Moran P, Borschmann R, Dean K, Hart C, Hogg J et al (2015) Domestic and sexual violence against patients with severe mental illness. Psychol Med 45(4):875–886
Khalifeh H, Oram S, Osborn D, Howard LM, Johnson S (2016) Recent physical and sexual violence against adults with severe mental illness: a systematic review and meta-analysis. Int Rev Psychiatry 28(5):433–451
Khawaja NG, White KM, Schweitzer R, Greenslade J (2008) Difficulties and coping strategies of Sudanese refugees: a qualitative approach. Transcult Psychiatry 45(3):489–512
Khadr S, Clarke V, Wellings K, Villalta L, Goddard A, Welch J et al (2018) Mental and sexual health outcomes following sexual assault in adolescents: a prospective cohort study. Lancet Child Adolesc Health 2(9):654–665
Kwankye SO, Richter S, Okeke-Ihejirika P, Gomma H, Obegu P, Salami B (2021) A review of the literature on

sexual and reproductive health of African migrant and refugee children. Reprod Health 18:1–13
Leamy M, Bird V, Le Boutillier C, Williams J, Slade M (2011) Conceptual framework for personal recovery in mental health: systematic review and narrative synthesis. Br J Psychiatry 199(6):445–452
Liu H, Petukhova MV, Sampson NA, Aguilar-Gaxiola S, Alonso J, Andrade LH et al (2017) Association of DSM-IV posttraumatic stress disorder with traumatic experience type and history in the World Health Organization World Mental Health Surveys. JAMA Psychiatr 74(3):270–281
MacMillan HL, Fleming JE, Streiner DL, Lin E, Boyle MH, Jamieson E et al (2001) Childhood abuse and lifetime psychopathology in a community sample. Am J Psychiatry 158(11):1878–1883
McCann TV, Mugavin J, Renzaho A, Lubman DI (2016) Sub-Saharan African migrant youths' help-seeking barriers and facilitators for mental health and substance use problems: a qualitative study. BMC Psychiatry 16:1–10
Miller KE, Rasmussen A (2010) War exposure, daily stressors, and mental health in conflict and post-conflict settings: bridging the divide between trauma-focused and psychosocial frameworks. Soc Sci Med 70(1):7–16
Mohammadifirouzeh M, Oh KM, Basnyat I, Gimm G (2023) Factors associated with professional mental help-seeking among US immigrants: a systematic review. J Immigr Minor Health 25(5):1118–1136
National Institute for Health and Care Excellence (2016) Domestic violence and abuse. Retrieved from: https://www.nice.org.uk/guidance/qs116/resources/domestic-violence-and-abuse-pdf-75545301469381
Nellums LB, Rustage K, Hargreaves S, Friedland J, Miller A, Hiam L (2018) Access to healthcare for people seeking and refused asylum in Great Britain: a review of evidence. Equality and Human Rights Commission
O'Doherty L, Whelan M, Carter GJ, Brown K, Tarzia L, Hegarty K et al (2023) Psychosocial interventions for survivors of rape and sexual assault experienced during adulthood. Cochrane Database Syst Rev 10(10). https://doi.org/10.1002/14651858.CD013456.pub2
O'Doherty L, Carter G, Sleath E, Brown K, Brown S, Lutman-White E, Jackson L, Heron J, Tek Kalsi P, Ladeinde OC, Whitfield D, Caswell R, Gant M, Halliwell G, Patel R, Feder G (2024) Health and well-being of survivors of sexual violence and abuse survivors attending sexual assault referral centres in England: the MESARCH mixed-methods evaluation. Health Soc Care Deliv Res 2024;12(35). https://doi.org/10.3310/CTGF3870
Oram S (2019) Sexual violence and mental health. Epidemiol Psychiatr Sci 28(6):592–593. https://doi.org/10.1017/S2045796019000106
Oram S, Abas M, Bick D, Boyle A, French R, Jakobowitz S et al (2016) Human trafficking and health: a survey of male and female survivors in England. Am J Public Health 106(6):1073–1078
Oram S, Khalifeh H, Howard LM (2017) Violence against women and mental health. Lancet Psychiatry 4(2):159–170. https://doi.org/10.1016/S2215-0366(16)30261-9
Ottisova L, Hemmings S, Howard LM, Zimmerman C, Oram S (2016) Prevalence and risk of violence and the mental, physical and sexual health problems associated with human trafficking: an updated systematic review. Epidemiol Psychiatr Sci 25(4):317–341
Pertek S, Phillimore J, Goodson L, Stevens A, Thomas S, Hassan P, Darkal H, Taal S, Altaweel R (2021) Forced migration and sexual and gender-based violence: findings from the SEREDA project in the UK. Research Report. University of Birmingham. Retrieved from: https://www.birmingham.ac.uk/Documents/college-social-sciences/social-policy/iris/2021/sereda-full-report.pdf
Phillimore J, Pertek S, Akyuz S, Darkal H, Hourani J, McKnight P et al (2022) "We are forgotten": forced migration, sexual and gender-based violence, and coronavirus disease-2019. Violence Against Women 28(9):2204–2230
Rosenberg M, Townes A, Taylor S, Luetke M, Herbenick D (2019) Quantifying the magnitude and potential influence of missing data in campus sexual assault surveys: a systematic review of surveys, 2010–2016. J Am Coll Heal 67(1):42–50
Ryan DA, Kelly FE, Kelly BD (2009) Mental health among persons awaiting an asylum outcome in Western countries: a literature review. Int J Ment Health 38(3):88–111
Şenses N (2020) Gender, women and precarity: examples from Turkey. In: Williams L (ed) Women, migration and asylum in Turkey: developing gender sensitivity in migration research, policy and practice. Palgrave Macmillan, pp 49–67. https://doi.org/10.1007/978-3-030-28887-7
Steine IM, Harvey AG, Krystal JH, Milde AM, Grønli J, Bjorvatn B et al (2012) Sleep disturbances in sexual abuse victims: a systematic review. Sleep Med Rev 16(1):15–25
Sweeney A, Clement S, Filson B, Kennedy A (2016) Trauma-informed mental healthcare in the UK: what is it and how can we further its development. Ment Health Rev J 21(3):174–192
Tarzia L, Thuraisingam S, Novy K, Valpied J, Quake R, Hegarty K (2018) Exploring the relationships between sexual violence, mental health and perpetrator identity: a cross-sectional Australian primary care study. BMC Public Health 18:1–9
United Nations (2024) Conflict-related sexual violence. Report of the United Nations Secretary General. Retrieved from: https://www.un.org/sexualviolenceinconflict/wp-content/uploads/2024/05/SG-2023-annual-reportsmallFINAL.pdf
UN Women (2016) The economic costs of violence against women. Retrieved from: https://www.unwomen.org/en/news/stories/2016/9/speech-by-lakshmi-puri-on-economic-costs-of-violence-against-women

Villalta L, Khadr S, Chua KC, Kramer T, Clarke V, Viner RM et al (2020) Complex post-traumatic stress symptoms in female adolescents: the role of emotion dysregulation in impairment and trauma exposure after an acute sexual assault. Eur J Psychotraumatol 11(1):1710400

Virupaksha HG, Kumar A, Nirmala BP (2014) Migration and mental health: an interface. J Nat Sci Biol Med 5(2):233–239. https://doi.org/10.4103/0976-9668.136141

Watters C (2001) Emerging paradigms in the mental health care of refugees. Soc Sci Med 52(11):1709–1718

Wirtz AL, Glass N, Pham K, Aberra A, Rubenstein LS, Singh S, Vu A (2013) Development of a screening tool to identify female survivors of gender-based violence in a humanitarian setting: qualitative evidence from research among refugees in Ethiopia. Confl Heal 7:1–14

World Health Organisation (2013) Responding to intimate partner violence and sexual violence against women: WHO clinical and policy guidelines. Retrieved from Geneva: http://apps.who.int/iris/bitstream/10665/85240/1/9789241548595_eng.pdf

World Health Organisation (2021) Violence against women prevalence estimates, 2018: global, regional and national prevalence estimates for intimate partner violence against women and global and regional prevalence estimates for non-partner sexual violence against women. Retrieved from: https://prevention--collaborative.org/wp-content/uploads/2021/08/WHO_2021_VAW-Estimates.pdf

World Health Organisation (2022) Refugee and migrant health. Retrived from: https://www.who.int/news-room/fact-sheets/detail/refugee-and-migrant-health

WRC (2016) A girl no more: the changing norms of child marriage in conflict. Women's Refugee Commission Retrieved from: https://www.womensrefugeecommission.org/wp-content/uploads/2020/04/Changing-Norms-of-Child-Marriage-in-Conflict.pdf

Advancing an Understanding of Relational Contexts of Depression with Urban Refugee Youth in Kampala, Uganda

7

Zerihun Admassu, Frannie MacKenzie, Carmen H. Logie, Moses Okumu, Robert Hakiza, Brenda Katisi, and Peter Kyambadde

Contents

Z. Admassu (✉) · F. MacKenzie
Factor-Inwentash Faculty of Social Work, University of Toronto, Toronto, ON, Canada
e-mail: zerihun.admassu@utoronto.ca; frannie.mackenzie@utoronto.ca

C. H. Logie
Factor-Inwentash Faculty of Social Work, University of Toronto, Toronto, ON, Canada

United Nations University Institute for Water, Environment, and Health, Hamilton, ON, Canada

Centre for Gender & Sexual Health Equity, Vancouver, BC, Canada

Women's College Research Institute, Women's College Hospital, Toronto, ON, Canada
e-mail: carmen.logie@utoronto.ca

M. Okumu
School of Social Work, University of Illinois at Urbana Champaign, Urbana, IL, USA

School of Social Sciences, Uganda Christian University, Mukono, Uganda
e-mail: okumu@illinois.edu

R. Hakiza · B. Katisi
Young African Refugees for Integral Development, Kampala, Uganda
e-mail: robert@yarid.org

P. Kyambadde
Most at Risk Population Initiative (MARPI), Kampala, Uganda

V. Padovese, I. Rossoni (eds.), *Intersections of Sexual Health, Migration and Sexualised Violence*, Sustainable Development Goals Series, https://doi.org/10.1007/978-3-032-20707-4_7

Abstract

Intimate partner violence (IPV) is linked to depression and disparities in sexual relationship power; gaining a deeper understanding of the pathways that underpin this relationship can enhance the development of targeted interventions for both relationship dynamics and depression. Both IPV and depression disproportionately affect refugees and require urgent attention, particularly among youth who are at a key development phase. As IPV can have long-lasting negative health impacts, reducing IPV risk and experiences is critical for long-term physical, mental, and sexual well-being. This is particularly salient among refugee youth, as experiences of IPV are more common compared with non-refugee counterparts and have been linked to depression. To deepen the understanding of these links, we explored the associations between intimate partner violence and depression and examined the mediation effects of sexual relationship power, referring to relational power dynamics and sexual decision-making. Cross- sectional data was collected from 346 urban refugee youth in Kampala, and structural equation modelling was used to test relationships between depression, IPV, and sexual relationship power. Results indicated that sexual relationship power, measured by the relationship control subscale, mediated the relationship between IPV and depression. IPV had direct ($\beta = 0.16$, $p = 0.002$, 95% CI: 0.06, 0.26) and indirect ($a\beta = 0.045$, $p = 0.004$, 95% CI: 0.014, 0.076) effects on depression.

These findings suggest that IPV both directly affects depression and reduces sexual relationship power that in turn also contributes to depression. It further underscores the urgent need for IPV prevention and gender-based violence prevention, as well as the integration of sexual relationship empowerment within larger programming for promoting healthy relationships and mental health.

Keywords

Intimate partner violence · Sexual relationship power · Depression · Youth refugees · Empowerment

7.1 Introduction

It is estimated that a third of women have experienced intimate partner violence at least once in their lifetime (World Health Organization 2021). Intimate partner violence refers to physical, sexual, or psychological behaviours by a current or previous intimate partner that cause harm and can result in long-term negative impacts on the health and well-being of those affected (World Health Organization 2021, 2022). Survivors of intimate partner violence (IPV) are nearly twice as likely to experience sexual and reproductive health problems, have poor general health, and engage in practices that might increase the likelihood of adverse health outcomes (World Health Organization 2022). While the negative health impacts of IPV are vast, it is critical to note the profound effect on mental health and well-being. The mental toll of IPV is significant, as those who experience it are nearly three times as likely to develop mental and neurological disorders (World Health Organization 2022). Further, IPV has been linked to depression, anxiety, and post-traumatic stress disorder, and a ten-times greater likelihood of attempting suicide than those not exposed (Lagdon et al. 2014; Potter et al. 2021).

It is pertinent to acknowledge the connection between IPV and mental health challenges among refugee youth, as they are at a disproportionate risk for both IPV victimization and mental health challenges (World Health Organization 2021, 2022; Logie et al. 2019; Dangmann et al. 2022). Refugees and displaced peoples face food insecurity, poverty, disruption of family and gender roles that can cause stress and exacerbate inequitable relationship power dynamics, and trauma that can result in substance use-related coping and reduced social support, all of which are risk factors for IPV (Logie et al. 2019; UNHCR 2003). One study found that more than 85% of urban refugee youth in an intimate relationship in Uganda had experienced IPV, which had direct effects on depression (Logie et al. 2019, 2020).

Although the risk of IPV is sixfold higher for refugee adults globally when compared to non-refugees (World Health Organization 2022), having higher sexual relationship power may mitigate the risks of IPV among refugee youth (Logie et al. 2019). Relationship power refers to the comparative level of control, independence, and ability to make decisions in a relationship (Blanc 2001). Imbalances in relationship power can influence sexual decision-making and limit the ability for those with lesser power to negotiate engagement in safer sexual practices (Closson et al. 2019). Sexual power imbalances can be influenced by a range of socio-cultural and economic factors. One of the major drivers is gender inequity, where traditional norms often grant men more control in sexual and relationship decisions. Young women, particularly in relationships with older men, face heightened vulnerability due to limited decision-making power and economic dependence (Closson et al. 2019, 2022). Gender-related social norms and expectations, such as patriarchal norms, further exacerbate these imbalances. Displacement adds additional household pressure as refugees often lose traditional support systems, intensifying women's reliance on male partners and increasing the risk of IPV (Roupetz et al. 2020). Disparities in sexual relationship power are associated with an elevated risk of IPV, particularly in contexts where one partner exerts disproportionate control over sexual decision-making (Closson et al. 2019, 2022). This is particularly salient among refugee youth, as relationship power imbalances may emerge from challenges such as language barriers, economic insecurity and the cultural assimilation that comes with migration (Hilsdon and Rozario 2006).

Understanding the role sexual relationship empowerment plays in the relationship between IPV and depression among refugee youth could influence interventions to reduce IPV, improve relationship power balance, and promote mental health. To deepen this understanding, we explored the mediation effects of sexual relationship power in relation to the associations between intimate partner violence and depression among urban refugee youth in Uganda among displaced and refugee youth living in five informal settlements (Nsambya, Katwe, Kabalagala, Kansanga, and Rubaga) in Kampala, Uganda, between 2021 and 2022. Rates of intimate partner violence (IPV) and depression are particularly high in Uganda's informal settlements, where these issues are compounded by socio-economic instability and displacement (Logie et al. 2020, 2022). Refugee and displaced populations are disproportionately affected by these challenges, which are intensified by the precarious living conditions and limited access to support services (Logie et al. 2019).

Specifically, we enrolled adolescents in a community-based cohort study aged 16–24 who self-identified as either refugees, displaced persons, or children of refugee/displaced parents. After obtaining informed consent, trained peer research assistants (PRAs) administered the surveys, ensuring confidentiality, offering counselling, and emphasizing that participants could skip any questions they found uncomfortable. Given the sensitive nature of topics, participants were provided with appropriate support and resources as needed. Participants were recruited using peer-driven and peer network sampling methods, which are particularly suited to reaching vulnerable and hard-to-access populations in these settings. The study received research ethics approval from the University of Toronto, Canada, and the Ugandan Ministry of Health.

7.2 Refugee Youth Profile

The study sample is profiled in Table 7.1. Of the 346 participants, nearly half (n = 166, 48.0%) were cisgender men, 50.3% (n = 174) were cisgender women, and six participants (1.7%) were transgender. The mean age of study participants was 21.2 (±2.6), with an age range of 16 to 24 years. Most participants had some level of

Table 7.1 Characteristics of refugee youth in Uganda (n = 346)

Variable	Frequency n (%)
Gender	
Cisgender men	166 (48%)
Cisgender women	174 (50.3%)
Transgender	6 (1.7%)
Age (mean/SD)	21.2 (2.6)
Length of time in Uganda	
1–5 years	132 (38.2%)
6–10 years	125 (36.1%)
More than 10 years	89 (25.7%)
Highest level of education $^{n=5}$	
Less than secondary	101 (29.6%)
Some secondary	211 (61.9%)
Secondary+	29 (8.5%)
Have children	
No	303 (87.6%)
Yes	43 (12.4%)
Intimate partner violence (IPV) in the past 3 months	
Yes	25 (7.2%)
No	321 (92.8%)
Depression (mean/SD) $^{n=3}$	5.9 (5.8)
Depression symptom severity	
None/Minimal (0–4)	172 (50.2%)
Mild (5–9)	79 (23.0%)
Moderate (10–14)	60 (17.5%)
Severe (15–27)	32 (9.3%)
SRP (mean/SD) $^{n=15}$	45.6 (10.2)
Sexual Relationship Power Scale (SRPS)	
Low	122 (37.2%)
Moderate	107 (32.6%)
High	99 (30.2%)

IPV intimate partner violence, *SD* standard deviation, *M* mean, *SRP* sexual relationship power, *N* missing value

secondary education (61.9%), and one-quarter of participants (25.7%) had lived in Uganda for less than 10 years. Twelve percent of the study participants had children ($n = 43$), with an average of 1.5 children. Participants reported ($n = 25$; 7.2%) having experienced intimate partner violence in the past 3 months. Nearly a quarter of participants (23.0%) reported mild depression, 17.5% reported moderate depression, and 9.3% reported severe depression. A third of the participants (32.6%) reported a moderate level of sexual relationship power, almost similar number (30.2%) reported a high level of sexual relationship power, and the highest number (37.2%) reported a low level of sexual relationship power.

7.3 Correlations Between Intimate Partner Violence, Sexual Relationship Power, and Depression

Means, standard deviations, and correlations between intimate partner violence, sexual relationship power, and depression are presented in Table 7.2. Mean scores for sexual relationship power and depression were 45.56 (SD = 10.25) and 5.91 (SD = 5.80), respectively. We found that intimate partner violence victimization was positively associated with higher levels of depression ($r = 0.22$, $p < 0.001$) and negatively associated with sexual relationship power ($r = -0.25$, $p < 0.001$) (Table 7.2). This means that participants reporting intimate partner violence had

Table 7.2 Mean, standard deviation of the variable and correlation between variables in the study

Variable	% (n)	M (SD)	IPV	SRP	Depression
IPV	7.23 (25)		–	−0.25**	0.22**
SRP		45.56 (10.25)	–	–	–
Depression		5.91 (5.80)	–	−0.27**	–

IPV intimate partner violence, *SD* standard deviation, *M* mean, *SRP* sexual relationship power lower sexual relationship power and higher depression scores.

7.4 Sexual Relationship Power Mediated the Effects of Intimate Partner Violence on Depression

Consistent with the proposed hypothesis, there were statistically significant associations for all pathways of the mediation model (Table 7.3). Results showed a direct significant association between intimate partner violence and depression ($\beta = 0.16$, $p = 0.002$, 95% CI: 0.06–0.26), with higher levels of IPV associated with higher levels of depression. Depression increased by 0.16 standardized unit for persons reporting intimate partner violence victimization compared with those who did not experience any intimate partner violence while adjusting for age and gender. There was also a significant negative correlation between sexual relationship power and depression ($\beta = -0.19$, $p < 0.001$, 95% CI: −0.30, −0.079), with lower sexual relationship power associated with higher levels of depression. Furthermore, there was a significant association between intimate partner violence and sexual relationship power ($\beta = -0.24$, $p = 0.002$, 95% CI: −0.34, −0.14), with more IPV exposure associated with less sexual relationship power (Table 7.3).

This analysis allowed us to examine whether intimate partner violence is associated with depression and whether this relationship is accounted for by sexual relationship power as a mediator. We found a significant indirect effect of intimate partner violence on depression through sexual relationship power (aβ = 0.045, $p = 0.004$, 95% CI: 0.014, 0.076). This means that higher intimate partner violence was associated with lower relationship power, which in turn was associated with higher depression (Table 7.3). Based on the Baron and Kenny approach (Baron and Kenny 1986), this finding establishes a partial mediation of intimate partner violence victimization through sexual relationship power to affect depression. About 22% of the effect of intimate partner violence on depression was mediated by sexual relationship power, suggesting that there were other mechanisms besides sexual relationship power that linked intimate partner violence and depression. A Sobel test was also conducted to test the hypothesized mediational model, to assess whether indirect effects were significant or not. The results showed that the complete pathway from intimate partner violence (independent variable) to sexual relationship power (mediator variable) to depression (dependent variable) was significant ($z = 2.858$, $p = 0.004$). This finding also supports that the sexual relationship power partially mediates the effects of intimate partner violence on depression (Table 7.4).

Table 7.3 Summary of structural equation modelling of the mediation model

Standardized	Coefficient	OIM std. err.	Z	$P > z$	95% conf. interval
Structural					
Sexual relationship power					
Intimate partner violence	−0.2364772	0.0506081	−4.67	0.000	−0.3356672, −0.1372872
Age	−0.1576403	0.0533388	−2.96	0.003	−0.2621823, −0.0530982
Gender	−0.0762336	0.0538559	−1.42	0.157	−0.1817892, 0.0293219
Depression					
Sexual relationship power	−0.1916386	0.053048	−3.61	0.000	−0.2956108, −0.0876665
Intimate partner violence	0.1572372	0.0520076	3.02	0.002	0.0553042, 0.2591702

Table 7.4 Significance testing of indirect effect (standardized)

Estímate	Delta	Sobel	Monte Carlo
Indirect effect	0.045	0.045	0.045
Std. Err.	0.016	0.016	0.017
z-value	2.838	2.858	2.734
p-value	0.005	0.004	0.006
Conf. Interval	0.014, 0.077	0.014, 0.076	0.017, 0.081

7.5 Discussion

The present study explored the association between intimate partner violence and depression, with the aim of examining whether sexual relationship power measured by relationship control subscale could be a potential mediator among urban refugee youth living in informal settlements in Uganda. Consistent with past research, our study found that young refugees who reported intimate partner violence also reported less power in their sexual relationships and increased depression. Furthermore, we found that the effect of intimate partner violence victimization on depression was partially mediated by sexual relationship power. The relationship between intimate partner violence and elevated levels of depression is complex, influenced by biochemical, psychological, and environmental risk factors that contribute to ongoing mental health challenges in survivors of abuse (Delara 2016), and our findings advance understanding of relationship power as an important factor to consider in this relationship.

Our findings align with previous studies indicating that depression is a critical mental health concern in interventions for addressing intimate partner violence among adolescents in informal settings (Logie et al. 2019; Bacchus et al. 2018). For instance, a study in informal settlements in South Africa found that participants experiencing IPV reported greater depressive symptoms (Gibbs et al. 2018), while research in rural Rwanda demonstrated a reciprocal relationship between IPV and depression (Chatterji and Heise 2021). This study further confirms and extends existing evidence that survivors of intimate partner violence report a lack of power in their relationships, and diminished relationship power is a risk factor for violence (Hulley et al. 2023).

The observed associations are consistent with disempowerment theory (Archer 2022; Gelles 1999), which suggests that a range of individual and intimate relationship risk factors predict the use of violence to re-establish power in a relationship. For instance, a study conducted in a Kenyan informal settlement reported that complex power dynamics contribute to an environment conducive to both IPV and HIV acquisition risks, particularly regarding women's lack of social and economic independence (Ringwald et al. 2023). Furthermore, rates of dating violence are significantly higher in relationships lacking shared power and decision-making (Felson and Messner 2000), and these barriers disproportionately affect minority, gender diverse, and immigrant youth (Kubicek 2018; Walters and Lippy 2016).

Future longitudinal studies should examine power differences between partners as potential predictors of intimate partner violence across gender and sexual orientation.

Perceived relationship power was significantly and negatively associated with depression in adjusted analyses, extending existing research that identifies an inverse relationship between sexual relationship power and depression (Filson et al. 2010; Hatcher et al. 2012; Minieri et al. 2014) to urban refugee youth in Kampala. Past research with non-refugee women in rural Uganda found that women with higher sexual relationship power experienced reduced depression symptom severity and better mental health compared to those with lower power (Hatcher et al. 2012). An imbalance of power can foster abusive behaviour and perpetuate a cycle of violence, negatively affecting the survivor's mental health and contributing to feelings of helplessness, low self-esteem, and increased vulnerability to mental health problems (La Flair et al. 2012). This relationship aligns with the "Gender and Power" theory, which suggests that unequal power dynamics hinder women's ability to exercise control in relationships (Maharaj 1995). Additionally, our findings resonate with the traumatic stress mechanism theory (Miller and Seligman 1975), where negative experiences, such as intimate partner violence, trigger biological stress responses that can affect mental health. This leads to significant psychological distress and challenges in coping, ultimately resulting in diminished power, self-esteem, and hope for the future and increased depressive symptoms (Brar et al. 2020).

7.6 Conclusions

In conclusion, this study provides evidence that intimate partner violence and sexual relationship power are linked to depression with urban refugee youth in Kampala. Additionally, sexual relationship power partially mediates the relationship between intimate partner violence and depression. Further research is needed to explore this mediating relationship through longitudinal and gender-stratified analyses, which were not possible here due to the small sample size. We also recommend utilizing both subscales of sexual relationship power in future studies to replicate these findings.

These findings can inform practice and policymakers in developing youth-centred, youth-led, community-based interventions for intimate partner violence that are culturally and contextually tailored for urban refugees in Kampala's informal settlements. Future interventions may benefit from insights gained from research in South Africa, which identified key factors contributing to the ineffectiveness of youth-focused intimate partner violence programmes: lack of involvement from both young women and men, a focus on individual risk factors without addressing broader social and structural contexts, and insufficient consideration of changes in gender norms and relationships (Mannell et al. 2019).

A collaborative approach with local stakeholders, including refugee youth themselves, is key to ensuring relevance and empowerment in addressing intimate partner violence and relationship dynamics. Gender transformative approaches that increase awareness and self-assessment of sexual relationship power among young refugees can build the foundation for gender-based violence prevention, programming for healthy relationships, and opportunities for early intervention for mental health promotion. Approaches that examine the syndemic of co-occurring and interacting social inequities (Logie et al. 2022)—such as relationship violence—and mental health challenges are key to meet the complexity of lived experiences and health needs and priorities of urban refugee youth in Kampala.

References

Archer J (2022) Power and male violence. In: Male violence [Internet], 1st edn. Routledge, London. [cited 2023 Dec 20]. Available from: https://www.taylorfrancis.com/chapters/edit/10.4324/9781003342717-20/power-male-violence-john-archer

Bacchus LJ, Ranganathan M, Watts C, Devries K (2018) Recent intimate partner violence against women and health: a systematic review and meta-analysis of cohort studies. BMJ Open 8(7):e019995

Baron RM, Kenny DA (1986) The moderator-mediator variable distinction in social psychological research: conceptual, strategic, and statistical considerations. J Pers Soc Psychol 51(6):1173–1182

Blanc AK (2001) The effect of power in sexual relationships on sexual and reproductive health: an examination of the evidence. Stud Fam Plan 32(3):189–213

Brar SK, Beattie TSH, Abas M, Vansia D, Phanga T, Maseko B et al (2020) The relationship between intimate partner violence and probable depression among adolescent girls and young women in Lilongwe, Malawi. Glob Public Health 15(6):865–876

Chatterji S, Heise L (2021) Examining the bi-directional relationship between intimate partner violence and depression: findings from a longitudinal study among women and men in rural Rwanda. SSM-Mental Health 1:100038

Closson K, Dietrich JJ, Beksinska M, Gibbs A, Hornschuh S, Smith T et al (2019) Measuring sexual relationship power equity among young women and young men South Africa: implications for gender-transformative programming. PLoS One 14(9):e0221554

Closson K, Lee M, Gibbs A, Nicholson V, Gormley R, Parry R et al (2022) Sexual relationship power equity is associated with consistent condom use and fewer experiences of recent violence among women living with HIV in Canada. J Acquir Immune Defic Syndr 90(5):482

Dangmann C, Dybdahl R, Solberg Ø (2022) Mental health in refugee children. Curr Opin Psychol 48:101460

Delara M (2016) Mental health consequences and risk factors of physical intimate partner violence. Ment Health Fam Med 12:119–125

Felson RB, Messner SF (2000) The control motive in intimate partner violence. Soc Psychol Q 63(1):86–94
Filson J, Ulloa E, Runfola C, Hokoda A (2010) Does powerlessness explain the relationship between intimate partner violence and depression? J Interpers Violence 25(3):400–415
Gelles RJ (1999) What causes men's violence against women? In: What causes men's violence against women? [Internet]. SAGE Publications, Inc., Thousand Oaks, pp 36–48. [cited 2023 Dec 20]. Available from: https://sk.sagepub.com/books/what-causes-mens-violence-against-women/n4.xml
Gibbs A, Dunkle K, Jewkes R (2018) Emotional and economic intimate partner violence as key drivers of depression and suicidal ideation: a cross-sectional study among young women in informal settlements in South Africa. PLoS One 13(4):e0194885
Hatcher AM, Tsai AC, Kumbakumba E, Dworkin SL, Hunt PW, Martin JN et al (2012) Sexual relationship power and depression among HIV-infected women in rural Uganda. PLoS One 7(12):e49821
Hilsdon AM, Rozario S (2006) Special issue on Islam, gender and human rights. Women's Stud Int Forum 4(29):331–338
Hulley J, Bailey L, Kirkman G, Gibbs GR, Gomersall T, Latif A et al (2023) Intimate partner violence and barriers to help-seeking among Black, Asian, minority ethnic and immigrant women: a qualitative metasynthesis of global research. Trauma Violence Abuse 24(2):1001–1015
Kubicek K (2018) Setting an agenda to address intimate partner violence among young men who have sex with men: a conceptual model and review. Trauma Violence Abuse 19(4):473–487
La Flair LN, Bradshaw CP, Campbell JC (2012) Intimate partner violence/abuse and depressive symptoms among female health care workers: longitudinal findings. Womens Health Issues 22(1):e53–e59
Lagdon S, Armour C, Stringer M (2014) Adult experience of mental health outcomes as a result of intimate partner violence victimisation: a systematic review. Eur J Psychotraumatol 5(1):24794
Logie CH, Okumu M, Mwima S, Hakiza R, Irungi KP, Kyambadde P et al (2019) Social ecological factors associated with experiencing violence among urban refugee and displaced adolescent girls and young women in informal settlements in Kampala, Uganda: a cross-sectional study. Conflict Health 13(1):60
Logie CH, Okumu M, Mwima S, Hakiza R, Chemutai D, Kyambadde P (2020) Contextual factors associated with depression among urban refugee and displaced youth in Kampala, Uganda: findings from a cross-sectional study. Confl Heal 14(1):45
Logie CH, Okumu M, Malama K, Mwima S, Hakiza R, Kiera UM et al (2022) Examining the substance use, violence, and HIV and AIDS (SAVA) syndemic among urban refugee youth in Kampala, Uganda: cross-sectional survey findings. BMJ Glob Health 7(Suppl 5):e006583
Maharaj Z (1995) A social theory of gender: Connell's gender and power. Fem Rev 49(1):50–65
Mannell J, Willan S, Shahmanesh M, Seeley J, Sherr L, Gibbs A (2019) Why interventions to prevent intimate partner violence and HIV have failed young women in southern Africa. J Int AIDS Soc 22(8):e25380
Miller WR, Seligman ME (1975) Depression and learned helplessness in man. J Abnorm Psychol 84(3):228–238
Minieri AM, Staton-Tindall M, Leukefeld C, Clarke JG, Surratt HL, Frisman LK (2014) Relationship power as a mediator of intimate partner violence and mental health issues among incarcerated, substance-using women. Int J Offender Ther Comp Criminol 58(3):303–319
Potter LC, Morris R, Hegarty K, García-Moreno C, Feder G (2021) Categories and health impacts of intimate partner violence in the World Health Organization multi-country study on women's health and domestic violence. Int J Epidemiol 50(2):652–662
Ringwald B, Taegtmeyer M, Mwania V, Muthoki M, Munyao F, Digolo L et al (2023) Power and poverty: a participatory study on the complexities of HIV and intimate partner violence in an informal urban settlement in Nairobi, Kenya. Soc Sci Med 336:116247
Roupetz S, Garbern S, Michael S, Bergquist H, Glaesmer H, Bartels SA (2020) Continuum of sexual and gender-based violence risks among Syrian refugee women and girls in Lebanon. BMC Womens Health 20(1):176
UNHCR (2003) Sexual and gender-based violence against refugees, returnees and internally displaced persons: guidelines for prevention and response. [cited 2023 Dec 19]. Available from: https://digitallibrary.un.org/record/532805
Walters ML, Lippy C (2016) Intimate partner violence in LGBT communities. In: The Wiley handbook on the psychology of violence. Wiley Blackwell, Hoboken, NJ, pp 695–714
World Health Organization (2021) Violence against women prevalence estimates, 2018: global, regional and national prevalence estimates for intimate partner violence against women and global and regional prevalence estimates for non-partner sexual violence against women. [Internet]. Geneva. [cited 2023 Nov 29]. Available from: https://www.who.int/publications-detail-redirect/9789240022256
World Health Organization (2022) Violence Info – Intimate partner violence [Internet]. [cited 2023 Dec 15]. Available from: http://apps.who.int/violence-info/intimate-partner-violence

Health in Immigration Detention and Alternatives to Detention

8

Jozef Bartovic, Soorej Jose Puthoopparambil, Elina Steinerte, and Kari Pahlman

Contents

All views expressed in this chapter are personal views of authors.

The author (Jozef Bartovic) is a staff member of the World Health Organization. The author alone is responsible for the views expressed in this publication and they do not necessarily represent the views, decisions or policies of the World Health Organization.'

J. Bartovic
World Health Organization, Regional Office for Europe, Copenhagen, Denmark

S. J. Puthoopparambil (✉)
WHO Collaborating Centre on Migration and Health Data and Evidence, Global Health and Migration Unit, Department of Women's and Children's Health, Uppsala University, Uppsala, Sweden
e-mail: soorej.jose@uu.se

E. Ste'inerte
Member of the UN Subcommittee on Prevention of Torture (SPT) and former Chair and Member of the UN Working Group on Arbitrary Detention (WGAD), Geneva, Switzerland

K. Pahlman
University of Sydney, Sydney, Australia

V. Padovese, I. Rossoni (eds.), *Intersections of Sexual Health, Migration and Sexualised Violence*, Sustainable Development Goals Series, https://doi.org/10.1007/978-3-032-20707-4_8

Abstract

This chapter synthesises evidence on the health and well-being impacts of immigration detention, drawing primarily on the WHO *Country Implementation Guide on Addressing the Challenges in Immigration Detention, and Alternatives to Detention*, the WHO *World Report on the Health of Refugees and Migrants,* and a supplementary rapid literature review to provide a global perspective. This chapter highlights well-documented harms associated with immigration detention worldwide, including physical and mental health hazards and risks of sexual and gender-based violence. The chapter concludes by exploring alternatives to detention and strategies for reducing harm in this context.

Keywords

Immigration detention · Human rights · Health · Sexual violence · Gender-based violence · SOGIESC

8.1 Introduction and Context

Immigration detention refers to the confinement of individuals and deprivation of liberty for migration-related proceedings (WHO 2022a). Despite international legal instruments clearly stating that detention should be used as a last resort only, and the well-known negative impacts of detention on health and well-being, immigration detention is increasingly resorted to as a means to manage migration flows (Weiler et al. 2022). As highlighted by the United Nations Working Group on Arbitrary Detention (WGAD) (2019), there is a 'growing and preoccupying practice of administrative detention, notably for those seeking asylum'.

Countries around the world employ different terms to describe immigration detention, including for example, reception and identification centres, transit zones, holding centres, or immigration removal centres, among others (WHO 2022a). The type and use of detention, and the approaches adopted to manage detention centres also vary globally. For example, detention facilities differ in terms of whether they are partially open or closed, whether structures are permanent and purpose-built or temporary, and the extent to which private for-profit contractors may be used to run facilities (Turnbull 2017). They also vary in terms of the length of time in which people may be detained and the conditions of their confinement, and whether children, families, and other persons in situations of vulnerability are also detained (Turnbull 2017). Access to legal representation and the existence of monitoring and inspection mechanisms and judicial oversight, as well as accessibility of centres to human rights organisations, also significantly vary globally (Turnbull 2017; Grange 2013).

Immigration detention generally falls under administrative laws. Most commonly it is the detention of non-citizens while their identity documents are verified, while their migratory status is being resolved or in preparation for a deportation process (WHO 2022b). However, the increasing criminalisation of irregular migration and asylum seeking in many countries around the world have also led to the growing use of immigration detention, including as a tactic of deterrence or punishment, or both (WHO 2022a; Turnbull 2017; Canning 2019). This is seen, for example, in countries where national legislation and policies effectively enable a practice of de facto indefinite detention, as seen previously in Australia for example, where the average length of immigration detention as of 31 March 2023 was

732 days (Molnar 2020; Australian Government Department of Home Affairs 2023).[1,2] Other countries such as Canada[3] and the United Kingdom also do not have legislated maximum lengths for administrative immigration detention at the time of writing (Global Detention Project 2016; Molnar 2020; Silverman et al. 2022; Stirling-Cameron and Goldenberg 2022).

The harms associated with immigration detention on the health and well-being of refugees and migrants around the world are well documented, including with respect to sexual and gender-based violence. This chapter aims to provide an overview of such impacts in a global context. After a brief note on methodology, there follows three key sections. The first is an introduction to the international legal framework that applies to immigration detention and the right to health and security of person. The second section provides an overview of evidence as it relates to the physical and mental health effects of immigration detention. The final section then discusses alternatives to detention and strategies for harm reduction in this context.

8.2 Methods

This chapter is based primarily on the evidence presented in the WHO Country Implementation Guide on Addressing the Challenges in Immigration Detention and Alternatives to Detention (2022a). This guide is based on a 2021 scoping review of both peer-reviewed (n = 42) and grey literature (n = 219) as it relates to health and immigration detention in the WHO European Region. It is also based on WHO's first World Report on the Health of Refugees and Migrants (2022b) and supplemented with an additional rapid literature review so as to provide a global perspective.

8.3 International Human Rights Laws and Standards

The use of immigration detention is governed by various international and legal instruments and standards that relate to the rights of detainees, including asylum seekers and irregular migrants. This includes customary international law, as well as treaties and protocols which are binding on state parties where they have been ratified or acceded. At the international level, the right of everyone to liberty and security of person is reflected in, for example, the International Covenant on Civil and Political Rights (ICCPR, Article 9(1)), the Convention on the Rights of Persons with Disabilities (CRPD, Article 14(1)(a)), the Convention on the Rights of the Child (CRC, Article 37(b)), and the International Convention on the Protection of All Migrant Workers and Their Families (CMW, Article 16(1)), among others (UNHCR 2018). It must be recalled that the Universal Declaration of Human Rights (UDHR) also codifies this right in Article 3, preceded only by the right to equality (Article 1) and prohibition of discrimination (Article 2), indicative of the importance of the right. The Human Rights Committee clarifies that 'everyone' includes, among others, 'aliens, refugees and asylum seekers, stateless persons, [and] migrant workers' (UNHCR 2018). CCPR/C/GC/35 (Para 3). The right to personal liberty is further recognised explicitly by all regional human rights instruments: The European Convention on Human Rights (ECHR, Article 5), the American Convention on Human Rights (IACHR, Article 7), the African Charter on Human and People's Rights, (ACHPR, Article 6), and the Arab Charter on Human Rights (The

[1] Since 2017, the WGAD has adopted over twenty individual opinions on de facto indefinite immigration detention in Australia. Refer to Opinions: No. 28/2017; No. 42/2017; No. 71/2017; No. 20/2018; No. 21/2018; No. 50/2018; No. 74/2018; No. 1/2019; No. 2/2019; No. 74/2019; No. 35/2020; No. 70/2020; No. 71/2020; No. 72/2020; No. 17/2021; No. 68/2021; No. 69/2021; No. 28/2022; No. 32/2022; No. 33/2022; No. 42/2022; No. 69/202; No. 14/2023; No. 15/2023; and No. 44/2023.

[2] On 8 November 2023, the High Court of Australia ruled that indefinite immigration detention is unlawful where there is no prospect for deportation (see Case S28/2023, NZYQ v. Minister for Immigration, Citizenship and Multicultural Affairs & Anor).

[3] See also WGAD, Opinion 7/2019 at para 64. UN Doc A/HRC/WGAD/2019/7.

Arab Charter, Article 14) which attests to the universal recognition of the right to personal liberty.

However, the right to personal liberty is not an absolute right and the deprivation of liberty has always been a legitimate form of state control over those within its jurisdiction and is recognised as such by all international and regional human rights instruments. Nevertheless, because the right of the state to detain is an exception to the general right of liberty of person, the right of liberty is closely linked to the prohibition of arbitrary detention in international law, and the prohibition of arbitrary detention is also universal and absolute (Steinerte 2022). It is also important to underscore that recognising a particular detention as 'lawful' does not necessarily mean that it is not arbitrary. Indeed, for any deprivation of liberty to comply with international law, it must first of all be lawful which means that the deprivation of liberty must abide by the substantive and procedural rules of the domestic legislation.[4] However, even when it does abide by it can still be arbitrary in international law since '[T]he notion of "arbitrariness" not to be equated with "against the law", but must be interpreted more broadly to include elements of inappropriateness, injustice, lack of predictability and due process of law, as well as elements of reasonableness, necessity and proportionality'.[5] Turning this to the detention in the context of migration, it is therefore paramount that any such detention is not only prescribed by law, but it should be also legitimate, necessary, proportionate, subject to regular, periodic review, and based on individual assessment. It must only be used as a last resort and only once all other alternatives have been exhausted and be imposed for the shortest possible time. Indeed, international standards require that the length of detention should be established by law and may not be unlimited or excessive in length (UNHCR 2018).[6] Consequently, the practice of indefinite detention is therefore, by definition, arbitrary.

Furthermore, it is important to emphasise that the right to seek asylum must be respected at all times, and immigration detention must not be applied punitively in a way that criminalises and seeks to deter people, whether in terms of duration of detention or conditions to which people are subjected (UNHCR 2018).[7]

International human rights instruments and standards are clear in stating that immigration detention should not be used for people in situations of vulnerability. Such persons may include children, survivors of trauma, pregnant and nursing mothers, victims of trafficking, persons with disabilities or other physical or mental health needs, and elderly persons. That children in particular should not be detained for migration-related purposes (regardless of their migratory status or that of their parent/s) is also reflected specifically in instruments such as the CRC.[8] Globally, however, as of 2021, at least 77 countries allow the detention of children for immigration-related purposes (WHO 2022a). The need to end the detention of children in the migration context was highlighted in 2020 by the UNHCR as an 'outstanding challenge' in its final progress report on its global strategy (2014–2019) to support governments and end the detention of asylum seekers and refugees (UNHCR 2020). In this report, the UNHCR notes that despite substantial progress having been made by governments and partners toward ending the detention of children, particular challenges must still be overcome to end such detention indefinitely and globally. Such challenges relate to border practices and the use of detention in transit zones, inadequate assessment procedures, the differential treatment of adolescents, and the lack of capacity of alternative suitable care arrangements, among other issues.

[4]Human Rights Committee, General Comment No. 35. UN Doc. CCPR/C/GC/35 at para 11.

[5]Human Rights Committee, General Comment No. 35. UN Doc. CCPR/C/GC/35 at para 12.

[6]WGAD, Revised Deliberation No. 5 at paras 19, 25–27. UN Doc A/HRC/39/45 at Annex 1.

[7]See also WGAD, Revised Deliberation No. 5 at paras 14, 22–24. UN Doc A/HRC/39/45 at Annex 1.

[8]See also WGAD, Revised Deliberation No. 5 at paras 11, 40–42. UN Doc A/HRC/39/45 at Annex 1.

Where detention is used, in respect to all persons, conditions must be humane and dignified and most notably must never amount to a treatment prohibited by international law. Indeed, the UDHR (Article 5) and the ICCPR (Article 7) both state that no one is to be subjected to torture, or inhumane, cruel or degrading treatment or punishment. The ICCPR (Article 10(1)) specifically states that even those deprived of liberty 'shall be treated with humanity and with respect for the inherent dignity of the human person' (UNHCR 2018). Crucially, the detention of asylum seekers or other irregular migrants must not take place in facilities such as police stations, remand institutions, prisons, and other such facilities designed for those within the criminal justice system.[9]

Standards of accommodation and conditions of detention are also governed by international human rights standards. This includes instruments such as the Convention Relating to the Status of Refugees (1951 Refugee Convention) and its 1967 Protocol, the 1998 Guiding Principles of Internal Displacement, as well as guidelines such as the SPHERE Handbook and the UNHCR Handbook for Emergencies (Razum and Butenop 2022). As highlighted in the WHO Country Implementation Guide (2022a), those detained should have access to basic necessities and amenities, including ensuring facilities are safe and gender-sensitive in this regard. They should have healthy and culturally appropriate food, access to outdoor space and recreation, and the ability to practice their religion freely and safely. Those detained must also have access to means of communication, including to friends and relatives, as well as to external services as required. The right to health for all people, regardless of legal status and documentation, is also underscored by international human rights law, including the Universal Declaration of Human Rights (Article 25) and the International Covenant on Economic, Social and Cultural Rights (see General Comment No. 20). It is also important to recall the United Nations Standard Minimum Rules for the Treatment of Prisoners (the Nelson Mandela Rules)[10] which in Rule 24 state that '[P]risoners should enjoy the same standards of health care that are available in the community, and should have access to necessary health-care services free of charge without discrimination on the grounds of their legal status.' This means that the detainees in the criminal justice context are to benefit from the healthcare level available to the public in general, known as a principle of equivalence of care. While the Nelson Mandela Rules of course do not apply to those detained in the immigration context, the parallels between the deprivation of liberty situations and the applicable standards are plain to see.

8.4 Health Impacts of Detention

Despite such right to health enshrined in international legal instruments, the adverse impacts of immigration detention on refugees and migrants who are detained are extensive and well documented. Not only does the experience of detention often impact upon belonging and identity (Turnbull 2017), but it also can result in severe physical and mental health impacts (WHO 2022a).

The WHO Country Implementation Guide (2022a) provides a scoping review of health outcomes among refugees and migrants in immigration detention, noting, however, that the findings included are of course not necessarily representative of the situation of all facilities in any given country, or of the region generally. The evidence presented provides an overview of the prevailing health challenges associated with the detention of migrants and refugees, where evidence is available, as well as key the contributing factors. The WHO Country Implementation Guide (2022a) establishes that both quality of life and health are consistently poor in immigration detention settings and, moreover, it is the substandard conditions of the detention environment itself that constitutes the main risk factor for overall

[9] See also WGAD, Revised Deliberation No. 5 at paras 11, 40–42. UN Doc A/HRC/39/45 at para 44.

[10] A/RES/70/175

poor health outcomes of those in detention. The duration of detention is also an important factor. Indeed, while the general health status of migrants is generally found to be comparable to that of the local host population upon arrival, however, it declines with increasing duration of detention (WHO 2022a). Unless otherwise cited, the evidence presented is drawn from the WHO Country Implementation Guide (2022a), focused primarily on the WHO European Region.

With regard to communicable diseases, the evidence is mixed. However, there is evidence that conditions such as overcrowding and poor sanitary conditions place people at increased risk for contracting communicable diseases, predominately related to overcrowding and poor sanitary conditions. For example, issues of inadequate infection prevention and control protocols, lack of access to fresh air and ventilation, and poor nutrition are among the factors found to have contributed to the occurrence and transmission of various communicable diseases in detention settings. These include respiratory, dermatological, and digestive diseases, among others. Such heightened risks for communicable diseases were highlighted during the COVID-19 pandemic. In many instances, overcrowded facilities with limited capacity to practice appropriate physical distancing, insufficient personal protection equipment, and the movement of staff through different facilities are among some of the factors that contributed to COVID-19 outbreaks in various immigration detention centres. At the same time, the use of some measures during the pandemic to reduce transmission risk, such as increased isolation, was also in many cases reported to be harmful and disproportionate.

The evidence regarding immigration detention and non-communicable diseases in the European Region is limited, though there is some research from other parts of the world that chronic conditions such as diabetes and heart disease often worsen in detention (Hampton et al. 2022). However, there is greater evidence regarding physical injuries and abuses and traumatic events that occur while refugees and migrants are in detention facilities which is of significant concern. This includes evidence in some settings of increased risk for physical and sexual assault, which will be discussed further below. Substandard living conditions have also been attributed to conditions such as malnutrition and dehydration in some settings (Hampton et al. 2022).

Data on women's health and child health as it pertains to immigration detention specifically in the Region is also limited. This is potentially related to the lower proportion of women and families in closed detention settings. The evidence that is available, however, indicates that immigration detention is harmful to the physical and mental health of women. In some cases, it is reported that women may have higher level of mental health disorders compared to detained males, or the general population, for example. Pregnant or breastfeeding women are known to be at particular risk of harm, not least due to lack of adequate and appropriate nutrition in some detention settings (Lungu-Byrne et al. 2021). Research indicates that at times a clear lack of access to reproductive autonomy, no or disrupted maternity care, and delayed or insufficient medical care including for those with high-risk pregnancies have been reported, as well as instances where antenatal care guidelines are not followed appropriately (Hourani et al. 2021).

Evidence on the health impact of detention on children clearly indicates that detention can lead to poor physical health outcomes in children, including development delays, food regression, sleep problems, as well as exacerbation of prior health conditions. Research also shows that infants may not always receive necessary care, and medical needs at times have gone unidentified or unrecognised, or unaddressed. Instances where initial immunisations have been missed or delayed are also reported. However, most available literature is also focused on the mental health impacts of detention in this context, with evidence demonstrating that children experience greater negative health impacts than adults. Indeed, the deterioration in mental health has been found to be often be more severe in children than in adults and also appear to continue for children following release from detention. The impacts include various mental health disorders including depression, anxiety and post-traumatic stress reactions, as well as social withdrawal, damaged attachment relationships, among other things (Fazel et al. 2014; Wood 2018).

The mental health impacts of immigration detention more broadly are the most widely studied health aspect, and the prevalence and severity of poor mental health are greater among migrants in immigration detention when compared to similar migrant populations living in community settings. Studies have found high prevalence of depression (up to 74%), anxiety (up to 56%), and post-traumatic stress disorder (up to 46%) among adults in immigration detention across the European Region, Australia, and the United States. A trend toward increasing rates of psychiatric disorders among those detained in these settings have also been reported. Moreover, a range of symptoms have been reported including sleep disorders, loss of appetite, and headaches. Instances of self-harm and attempted suicide have also been frequently reported.

Key stressors in this context include uncertainty around the duration of detention and reasons for being detained, confusion related to legal and migration procedures, lack of autonomy and feelings of being treated unjustly, and being made to feel like a criminal. Issues of staff decency, perceived and experienced mistreatment from staff, safety threats, incidents of violence and assault, and feeling of not being able to report needs and incidents safely are also major stressors that contribute to mental health concerns in these settings and will be discussed below. Isolation, separation from family, lack of activities, and lack of proper support systems in place in detention settings are other major factors, as well as the often unsafe and substandard conditions experienced (Lungu-Byrne et al. 2021).

Indeed, evidence consistently demonstrates that the conditions in immigration detention centres are key contributing factors in creating and/or exacerbating both physical and mental health concerns experienced by refugees and migrants. Despite the clear stipulations in international law and guidelines as outlined earlier, immigration detention centres across the European Region and in other parts of the world are often described as prison-like (Peterie 2018). This is evident through features such as use of high security features, the carrying of weapons by staff, detainees being referred to by number rather than name, the use of body searches, and use of old prison buildings, where criminals are no longer imprisoned, as immigration detention facilities. Additionally, further curtailment of freedoms such as being locked in rooms at night, or being placed in isolation or solitary confinement also exist within detention (Bonfiglio et al. 2020). As previously mentioned, frequent complaints across many detention facilities also include inadequate food and nutrition, poor hygiene conditions such as bathroom facilities, overcrowding, etc. (Fazel et al. 2014; Lungu-Byrne et al. 2021). In another scoping review of environmental conditions in detention settings across the European region, it was found that conditions are often substandard, even when compared to prisons, and potentially in breach of human rights standards (Lungu-Byrne et al. 2021). Here, overcrowding and unsanitary conditions, lack of safe drinking water, and lack of safety and privacy were also highlighted as key environmental stressors (Lungu-Byrne et al. 2021).

Lack of provision of appropriate health care services in such settings contributes to poor health outcomes. The management and provision of health care services in immigration detention around the world vary; some countries specify the services available in national laws and regulations while others do not. Medical screening is often provided at the point of entry into a country and into detention facility, however, it is generally focused on communicable diseases. Indeed, screening practices in the European Region have seldom been found to be comprehensive, for example, failing to include mental health components. Lack of continuous health screening (and care) also remains an issue.

In the European Region, while essential and emergency care is generally provided in immigration detention facilities, access to secondary and tertiary specialised care services is frequently lacking. It is also reported that requests for care often go unheard or are not handled in a timely manner. This includes for routine concerns, such as accessing prescription medication. In other regions, such as in the United States, researchers have documented instances of medical neglect in various immigration detention settings, for example, withholding of essential medications that have resulted in severe harms, failing to administer routine vaccinations, or providing incomplete treatment regimes or not handling side effects or necessary specialist referrals appropriately or in a timely manner (Bonfiglio et al. 2020). Where detainees are released, doing so without appropriate follow-up where this is medically required is another example (Bonfiglio et al. 2020).

8.5 Sexual and Gender-Based Violence in the Detention Context

Immigration detention centres are sites where risks for sexual and gender-based violence are often heightened. Indeed, the perpetration of sexual and gender-based violence has been widely and increasingly documented in immigration detention settings worldwide (Kirby 2020; Tan and Kuschminder 2022; WHO 2022a; Freyer and McKay 2021; Lue et al. 2023). The lack and/or inadequacy of safety and protection measures within detention facilities contributes to increased risks, as well as instances where such violence may be systematically perpetrated, including as a form of torture (Kirby 2020). The scale of such, however, is difficult to estimate and the full extent of sexual and gender-based violence is unknown as cases are almost certainly underreported. This is likely owing to lack of meaningful access to reporting mechanisms in many instances, stigma, as well as fear of any consequences or retaliation from reporting, whether real or perceived (Ramsy 2021; Lue et al. 2023). There could also be instances where detainees do want to report such violence as the perpetrators might be part of the government agencies that are involved in the detention case. Even where cases are reported and allegations made, many are left uninvestigated, while the burden of proof placed on survivors can exacerbate their trauma (O'Leary 2019).

It is also important to note that many of those who are at risk for sexual and gender-based violence in detention settings may already be survivors of violence and trauma, having been likely exposed to such forms of violence during their journey through home, transit, and destination countries. For example, a study of asylum reception centres across seven European Union (EU) countries found that more than half of interviewed residents had experienced at least one instance of sexual and gender-based violence in the year prior (Oliveira et al. 2018; Tan and Kuschminder 2022). Another study of migrants in Belgium and the Netherlands again found that more than half had experienced such violence since arriving within the EU (Keygnaert et al. 2012; Tan and Kuschminder 2022). Experience of sexual and gender-based violence in third country transit zones is particularly common, with numerous reports of high rates of victimisation and systematic brutality occurring along migration routes through Libya, for example (e.g. Kirby 2020; Tan and Kuschminder 2022; Women's Refugee Commission 2019). The most commonly reported sexual violence occurs in the form of forced transactional sex and coercion, and as an element of forced labour and torture, among other forms, including as perpetrated by border authorities and local police, and in detention and reception centres by asylum professionals (Kirby 2020; Tan and Kuschminder 2022; Freedman et al. 2022). Sexual and gender-based violence in the form of intimate partner violence domestic violence also occurs along migratory routes (Tan and Kuschminder 2022). Importantly, it is not just women and girls at high risk for sexual and gender-based violence; studies show that in some migratory contexts, such violence perpetrated against men and boys can be just as widespread, if not more so (Tan and Kuschminder 2022). Members of the LGBTIQ+ community are also often at heightened risk for such violence and will be discussed in more detail below.

A similar picture emerges in other parts of the world. In the United States, scholars have described an 'epidemic' of sexual violence and abuse in immigration detention centres across the country (O'Leary 2019; Ramsy 2021; Lue et al.

2023).[11] In a study of sexual assault allegations perpetrated against individuals across 129 United States Immigration and Customs Enforcement (ICE) facilities between 2018 and 2022, it was found that more than 70% of facilities reported allegations, with the rate of sexual assault in detention occurring at a rate of up to 3.5 times higher than in the general population (Lue et al. 2023). O'Leary (2019) reports that the perpetration of sexual violence across the United States have typically been worst in those facilities that are privately operated. Investigations into reports of violence are also rare. In California, for example, O'Leary (2019) reports that between 2000 and 2016, there were 4500 complaints of sexual assault from within private facilities reported to the Department of Homeland Security Office of the Inspector General; only 1% of these were investigated. Indeed, sexual and gender-based violence is a common experience of many migrants in detention in the United States, and yet there is a reported 'system-wide unresponsiveness' to the issue (Ramsy 2021). Scholars have pointed to the myriad of structural barriers to accessing justice and redress, including lack of access to counsel and other meaningful legal resources or remedies for survivors (Ramsy 2021; O'Leary 2019). It is important to note that immigration detention can happen during any phase of the migratory journey—pre-departure, transit, arrival, or return (WHO 2022a). This also means that survivors of sexual violence can be detained and can be subjected to sexual violence while being detained as shown above.

The systematic and structural perpetration of sexual and gender-based violence is again prevalent in other parts of the world. In Australia, for example, sexual violence has similarly been documented as 'part of the repertoire of deterrence' and punishment in immigration detention centres (Perera and Pugliese 2021). Indeed, such violence is described in some cases as institutional, i.e. gendered harms as part of state-perpetrated violence against forced migrants (Hourani et al. 2021; Vasefi and Dehm 2022). Essex (2020) documents that such forms of violence has been common particularly since the beginning of 'offshore' detention practices, with reports of sexual and physical assault against migrants and refugees detains as also having been previously dismissed or covered up. Official reports, concluding from UNHCR and parliamentary inquiries, have outlined gender-specific harms related to offshore detention; instances of sexual assault and harassment for example have been documented in the Nauru detention centre, particularly against women but also children and youth (Rivas and Bull 2018; Freyer and McKay 2021; Passardi et al. 2022). In an analysis of 2116 publicly available incident reports from the detention centre in Nauru recorded between May 2013 and October 2015, including violations of the UDHR, Freyer and McKay (2021) found 748 related to breaches of Article 3 of the UDHR (right to life, liberty, and security), including sexual assault. These incidents were perpetrated by both other detainees, as well as centre security staff who in some cases were reported to be requesting sexual favours (Freyer and McKay 2021). Some incidents were also perpetrated against children and youth (Freyer and McKay 2021). Sexual and gender-based violence in this context can also be seen further in relation to infringements on the right to privacy, such as when showering or dressing; the lack of safe and appropriate facilities for women and girls within detention facilities in Australia have been highlighted (Freyer and McKay 2021; Vasefi and Dehm 2022).

Other examples of gendered violence in this context also include reproductive oppression and harm, and the violent treatment of pregnant migrants and mothers in detention. Again, in the United States for example, there are documented cases of not only physical violence against pregnant women, but clear instances of medical neglect and where request for medical attention go ignored (Heffernan 2023). This includes reported cases of stillbirths and miscarriages, and live births without medical attention (Heffernan 2023). Other examples have also been highlighted, such as being denied sufficient food, water, and items to keep warm (including for newborns), as well as having essential medications withheld or confiscated, and being subject

[11] See for example A/HRC/36/37/Add.2.

to medical procedures where they may not be necessary or consented to (Heffernan 2023). Barriers to accessing abortion in detention in the United States have been described as 'insurmountable' and the lack of social and material support generally has been documented (Heffernan 2023).

8.5.1 Sexual and Gender-Based Violence, and People of Diverse Sexual Orientation, Gender Identity and Expression, and Sex Characteristics (SOGIESC)

The risk of sexual and gender-based violence in immigration detention is particularly great for those already at heightened risk of discrimination, abuse, and exploitation. The International Detention Coalition (2016) reports that 'almost universally, LGBTQI+ persons are in situations of extreme vulnerability'. Indeed, as Kurdyla (2022) highlights, the intersection of sexual orientation and gender identity, and immigration status, may result in very different experiences of migration and detention for many, including with respect to exposure to sexual and gender-based violence. Some may be seeking asylum based on previous persecution due to their sexual orientation and/or gender identity, or they may be seeking asylum on other grounds or are otherwise migrants who left for other reasons and then are detained (Tabak and Levitan 2014). When in detention, however, LGBTQI+ people often face significantly increased vulnerability to human rights abuses, particularly if perceived as not conforming with prevailing social norms (Tabak and Levitan 2014; Kurdyla 2022). Indeed, non-conforming refugees and migrants with diverse SOGIESC are often exposed to sexual and gender-based violence, assault, harassment, and stigmatisation, both from other people are detained, and by detention staff and security (Tabak and Levitan 2014).[12] Transgender migrants and particularly transgender women are noted by some to be potentially at particularly high risk, for example, when placed in accommodation according to sex-assigned-at-birth, or in confinement, increasing risk of victimisation by other detainees or staff (Tabak and Levitan 2014; Kurdyla 2022). Specialised essential medical care for these groups, including often life-saving gender-affirming care, is in many instances lacking or denied entirely (Marquez-Velarde et al. 2023; Kurdyla 2022).

The in/visibility of refugees and migrants with diverse SOGIESC in immigration detention settings is an important and challenging issue. Indeed, while in some instances, there are protection measures in place for LGBTQI+ people within national migration and asylum systems[13], this generally requires self-identification, and where refugees and migrants do not publicly express their sexual orientation and gender identity, this may lead to critical protection gaps. At the same time, however, such public expression in many cases instead only leads to increased exposure to violence, harm, and discrimination (Tabak and Levitan 2014). Generally, protection mechanisms for LGBTQI+ refugees and migrants in many detention settings around the world are lacking, and available support services are often minimal. Thus, these groups are also often understood as being invisible to protection mechanisms within the migration and asylum processes—also due to the generally binary gender discourse within legal systems—at the same time making them hyper visible as they remain in situations where they may face constant risk of victimisation (Nematy et al. 2022; Kurdyla 2022; Tabak and Levitan 2014). This is also a concern related to those seeking asylum due to persecution related to their SOGIESC; that is, the inherent

[12] See for example A/HRC/36/37/Add.2 at para 34.

[13] In the European Region, for example, the recognition of LGBTQI+ persons as 'vulnerable' and therefore subject to particular protective measures is not consistent. Notably, the Common European Asylum System (CEAS) Directive 13/33/EU which sets out reception standard and protection guarantees for vulnerable persons (Chap. IV, Articles 21 and 22) does not specifically mention LGBTQI+ individuals. Scholars have pointed to this having significant potential to risk human rights protections regarding safe accommodation and access to necessary support services for these groups (Tschalaer 2023).

harm in needing to prove the credibility of one's claim while knowing that doing so can therefore increase vulnerability in detention contexts. Thus, LGBTIQ+ refugees and migrants, alongside other vulnerable groups, should not be placed in detention to the extent possible, but rather accommodated in facilities that meet their needs. The importance of exploring alternatives to detention will be discussed in the following section.

As the examples above highlight, immigration detention are sites of increased risk for sexual and gender-based violence. And, while certain groups such as women and girls, or LGBTIQ+ refugees and migrants are understood to be vulnerable throughout the processes of migration and displacement including in detention, it is important to note that it is also immigration-related policies and practices themselves that actively contribute to or increase vulnerability through risk of violence (Canning 2019). As Canning (2019) writes, reflecting on research conducted on the experiences of women in detention seeking asylum in the United Kingdom, Sweden, and Denmark, it is indeed the actions and inactions of the states that are bound by international law to protect them that make them *more* vulnerable, not less. It is clear that there are greater efforts needed to improve the safety and security of refugees and migrants in this context around the world. The following section provides a brief overview of strategies for harm reduction and the importance of utilising alternatives to detention where possible.

8.6 Harm Reduction and Alternatives to Detention

As stated by the Global Detention Project (2023), 'if a policy is inherently harmful, then there are arguably no "best practices" to promote, only harm reducing ones'. As highlighted earlier, international legal standards and guidelines clearly and unequivocally state that when there is a decision to detain an individual for migration-related reasons, alternatives to detention and non-custodial measures should be prioritised wherever possible that respect both the right to liberty and the right to health. Decisions should be based on individual assessment, and people in vulnerable situations should also never be detained. In effect, states should at all times opt for the least restrictive measures available and focus on promoting alternatives to detention (ATD) where possible. It is however crucial to recall that alternatives to detention should only be considered when all the requirements for detention have been satisfied in the first place. Therefore, consideration of alternatives to detention should never arise in respect to such vulnerable groups as children since international law prohibits their detention in the first place.

While the term 'alternatives to detention' is not a legal one, and there is no global consensus on the term, it is generally considered to refer to policies that enable refugees and migrants who would otherwise be detained to instead complete the administrative migration-related processes while residing within the community (WHO 2022a). There are a variety of ATD strategies employed throughout the Region and beyond, with different approaches applying more or less restrictions depending, so as to ensure compliance (WHO 2022a).

Indeed, ATD encompass both enforcement- and engagement-based approaches. As explained by the WHO Country Implementation Guide (2022a, b), enforcement approaches are those that still impose some restrictions on movement, yet do not constitute deprivation of liberty in the same way that immigration detention does. Engagement-based approaches meanwhile refers to methods that promote engagement and cooperation between refugees and migrants and the immigration system; they tend to be based in the community and provide case management based on trust. It is the later approach that should be prioritised to the extent possible, as supported by most UN relevant agencies and organisations (WHO 2022a).

Appropriate and effective use of alternatives can demonstrate respect for human rights while still meeting compliance with immigration procedures and can be cost effective to the state

(Council of Europe 2019; WHO 2022a). The Council of Europe (2019) has reported that alternatives are between twice and up to 17 times less expensive than detention. Critically, they are also generally better protection for people in vulnerable situations (Council of Europe 2019).

The COVID-19 pandemic demonstrated the various possibilities of realising alternatives to detention. Indeed, the risk for COVID-19 in many detention centres meant that the condition of proportionality that had to be met to justify continued detention no longer applied in the same way since the risk factors changed. Indeed, according to the WGAD, Detention in the context of migration is only permissible as an exceptional measure of last resort, which is a particularly high threshold to be satisfied in the context of a pandemic or other public health emergency.[14] As a result, in many jurisdictions, governments adopted measures that indicated the continued possibility of realising alternatives to detention. Such measures included release from detention, registration and support in the community, extension of residency permits, relaxation or cessation of reporting requirements, the use of firewalls for provision of health services, and non-discriminatory access to essential rights and services, among other things (Chew et al. 2020).

In addition to exploring and pursuing ATD, there are other important short- and medium-term actions and recommendations with respect to the use of detention, mitigating the negative impact of detention on health and preventing and responding to sexual and gender-based violence. Key areas for intervention across both state-run and privately operated facilities—based on the Ottawa Charter for Health Promotion (1086)—relate to building healthy public policies, creating supportive environments, strengthening community action, developing personal skills, and reorienting health services. Such recommended actions are highlighted in brief below.

[14]WGAD, Deliberation No. 11 on prevention of arbitrary deprivation of liberty in the context of public health emergencies, at para 24. UN Doc A/HRC/45/16, Annex II.

Healthy policies

- Develop and standardise legal obligations to examine the use of ATD in all possible instances; the use of immigration detention should be a last resort following individual assessment. Where the use of ATD is considered, there should still be a need and a legal basis, and it be proportionate to the individual circumstances present. Immigration detention for children is prohibited.
- Immigration detention should not be used for individuals in vulnerable situations. Vulnerability screening should be carried out for all individuals before entering detention and at regular intervals. Systems and/or processes should be established that trigger referrals where required and ensure appropriate support is provided.
- Strengthen the right to health and support systems for refugees and migrants in immigration detention, without discrimination. Those in immigration detention should have access to the same public health standards and protocols as implemented in the local community, and equivalence of care should be afforded, including during health emergencies.
- Data from immigration detention facilities should be systematically and safely collected and easily accessible, including the number of individuals in immigration detention, and enrolled in ATD.

Supportive environments

- Use only designated facilities for immigration detention; police stations should not be used, nor should refugees and migrants be placed in the same spaces as those in prisons. Any prison-like characteristics should be avoided.
- Address overcrowding in immigration detention, especially so as to reduce the risk of communicable disease transmission and minimise the impact on the mental health of those detained.
- Ensure provision of appropriate physical amenities, recreational space and meaningful activities, and nutritious and culturally and religiously appropriate food.

- Ensure specialised and appropriate care and accommodation is available and afforded to refugees and migrants in vulnerable situations, including those with diverse SOGIESC, as well as to pregnant women and girls and mothers that ensures availability and continuity of pre-and post-natal care. For refugees and migrants with disabilities, accommodations must also be accessible, and arrangements made so as to meet their specific needs.
- Gender-sensitive policies should be initiated, including with respect to the physical environment. This includes ensuring safe access to designated facilities and sanitary supplies for women and that privacy is afforded for undertaking personal activities. Physical and social safeguards should further be implemented and/or strengthened that focus on preventing sexual and gender-based violence and exploitation, including provision of protection and response mechanisms such as counselling and need-based health care and referral, where consented to.
- Improve integration of sexual and gender-based violence monitoring into detention monitoring and enforcement mechanisms. Reporting procedures should be clear, reliable, and safe, and all claims should be duly investigated by an independent authority in a timely manner.
- Access to confidential legal assistance must be available for all refugees and migrants in immigration detention.
- Communication methods should be appropriate, including providing information in languages understood by refugees and migrants, and using professional interpreters. Information should be provided on why they are being detained, expectations and available services, and length of stay, among other things.
- Sufficient resources should be provided to enable refugees and migrants to communicate with the outside world, including access to family and friends, and online resources.

Community actions

- Ensure coordination and networking between organisations to allow for the exchange of information and good practices. Create or strengthen working groups and committees comprising all stakeholders involved in supporting or interacting with refugees and migrants in immigration detention.
- Carry out regular, independent monitoring of conditions and treatment in immigration detention and ensure that appropriate solutions to issues are identified and implemented in a timely manner. Accountability mechanisms should be established to ensure issues and recommendations presented to migration authorities during monitoring visits are duly implemented, and relevant reports should be published and shared transparently. Collaborations between monitoring bodies and immigration detention bodies should also be implemented to facilitate the implementation of the recommendations.
- Strengthen the utilisation of community-based ATD and support models, including through supporting research on ATD and its impact on health and well-being to enable evidence-informed policymaking. Community resources and funding are needed to ensure that both human resources and services are sufficient to enable utilisation of ATD programs.

Developing personal skills

- Implement timely skill development for staff working in immigration detention on issues pertaining to human rights standards and legal responsibilities. This includes provision of non-discriminatory care for people with diverse SOGIESC, preventing and responding to sexual and gender-based violence, and upholding child protection measures, among other issues.
- Ensure training for all staff working in immigration detention includes first aid (including mental health first aid) and understanding of appropriate referral pathways. Support profes-

sional development to enhance cultural competencies of staff.
- Ensure support mechanisms are in place for all staff working in immigration detention to help them address the ethical concerns they may face during their work. Mental health and psychosocial support services should also be available to staff.

Appropriate health services
- Establish needs-based access to free health care for all refugees and migrants in immigration detention, at the earliest possible opportunity, and on an ongoing basis. Move refugees and migrants who require health care to appropriate facilities if such services are not available in immigration detention and establish strong referral pathways.
- Ensure health care providers have independence and autonomy in their practice and that priorities and responsibilities between health care providers and immigration detention staff are aligned to ensure timeliness and quality of care.
- Health screening should be systematically integrated in immigration detention so as to shift toward a preventative health-care model. Screening for physical and mental health should be provided upon entry to facilities, and regular assessments conducted. Ensure appropriate services are available for follow-up as required, and strengthen referral pathways between immigration detention facilities and local health systems.
- Continuity of care should be ensured though the use of robust reporting across community health care networks and within immigration detention.

8.7 Conclusions

The environment within immigration detention is a key risk factor for poor physical and mental health, including for sexual and gender-based violence. Despite such known harms, as well as clear requirement in international law that detention in migratory context be a measure of last resort and a clear prohibition to detain certain categories such as children, immigration detention continues to be used frequently as a migration management tool worldwide. Moreover, the conditions within immigration detention often do not reflect its intended administrative nature, with many facilities across the region and globally failing to adhere to the necessary safeguards and provisions as stipulated in international laws and guidelines. This chapter offers a useful summary of some of the key impacts of immigration detention on the health and well-being of refugees and migrants, highlighting in particular the epidemic of violations of sexual and reproductive rights within many immigration detention facilities globally. The international community must take timely action by prioritising alternatives to detention to the extent possible and minimising harm where it may arise. Key opportunities for intervention include building healthy public policies, creating supportive environments, strengthening community action, developing personal skills, and reorienting health services appropriately. Such actions are essential to ensure that the health and human rights of all persons, including refugees and migrants, are upheld in accordance with international law and in the spirit of equity, solidarity, and humanity. They are also paramount to give real meaning to the requirement of international law that detention is an exceptional measure in the migratory context.

References

Australian Government Department of Home Affairs (2023) Immigration detention and community statistics summary: March 2023. Available at: https://www.homeaffairs.gov.au/research-and-stats/files/immigration-detention-statistics-31-march-2023.pdf

Bonfiglio G, Rosal K, Henao-Martinez A, Franco-Paredes C, Poeschla EM, Moo-Young J, Seefeldt T, Dunlevy H, Haas M, Young J (2020) The long journey inside immigration detention centres in the USA. J Travel Med 27(7):2020

Canning V (2019) Degradation by design: women and asylum in northern Europe. Race Class 61(1):46–63

Chew V, Phillips M, Yamada Park M (2020) COVID-19 impacts on immigration detention: global responses. International Detention Coalition and HADRI/Western Sydney University

Council of Europe (2019) Practical guidance on alternatives to immigration detention: fostering effective results. Available at: https://rm.coe.int/migration-practical-guide-alternatives-migration/1680990236

Essex R (2020) The healthcare community and Australia immigration detention: the case for non-violent resistance. Palgrave Macmillan, Singapore

Fazel M, Karunakara U, Newnham EA (2014) Detention, denial, and death: migration hazards for refugee children. Lancet Glob Health 2(6):e313–e314

Freedman J, Sahraoui N, Tastsoglou E (eds) (2022) Gender-based violence in migration: interdisciplinary, feminist and intersectional approaches. Palgrave Macmillan

Freyer B, McKay FH (2021) An investigation of incident reports from the detention Centre Nauru: has Australia breached the Universal Declaration of Human Rights? J Human Rights 20(4):449–467

Global Detention Project Annual Report (2016) Global Detention Project | Mapping immigration detention around the world. Available online. Last accessed 13 May 2026

Global Detention Project (2023) Building partnerships, harnessing data, ending arbitrary immigration detention: Annual report 2023. Available at: https://www.globaldetentionproject.org/2022-annual-report-building-partnerships-harnessing-data-ending-arbitrary-immigration-detention

Grange M (2013) Smoke screens: is there a correlation between migration euphemisms and the language of detention? Global Detention Project Working Paper 5:1–11

Hampton K, Mishori R, Griffin M, Hillier C, Pirrotta E, Wang NE (2022) Clinicians' perceptions of the health status of formerly detained immigrants. BMC Public Health 22:575

Heffernan A (2023) Pregnancy in the United States immigration detention: the gendered necropolitics of reproductive oppression. Int Fem J Polit 25(1):30–53

Hourani J, Block K, Phillimore J et al (2021) Structural and symbolic violence exacerbates the risks and consequences of sexual and gender-based violence for forced migrant women. Front Hum Dyn 3. https://doi.org/10.3389/fhumd.2021.769611

International Detention Coalition (2016) LGBTI persons in immigration detention: position paper. Available at: https://idcoalition.org/wp-content/uploads/2016/06/LGBTI-Position_web_June-2016.pdf

Keygnaert I, Vettenberg N, Temmerman M (2012) Hidden violence is silent rape: sexual and gender-based violence in refugees, asylum seekers and undocumented migrants in Belgium and The Netherlands. Cult Health Sex 14(5):505–520

Kirby P (2020) Sexual violence in the border zone: the EU, the women, peace and security agenda and carceral humanitarianism in Libya. Int Aff 96(5):1209–1226

Kurdyla V (2022) Advocating for transgender immigrants in detention centres: cisnormativity as a tool for racialized social control. Am Behav Sci 66(13):1777–1796

Lue N, Nwadiuko J, Parmar P, Zeidan A (2023) Trends in sexual assault against detainees in US immigration detention centres, 2018-2022. JAMA J Am Med Assoc 329(4):338–339

Lungu-Byrne C, Germain J, Plugge E, van Hout MC (2021) Contemporary migrant health experience and unique health care needs in European prisons and immigration detention centres. Int J Forensic Ment Health 20(1):80–99

Marquez-Velarde G, Miller GH, Marquez BA, Shircliff JE, Suárez MI (2023) Transgender in detention: victimization experiences in immigration facilities. Transgender Health. preprint. https://doi.org/10.1089/trgh.2022.0083

Molnar P (2020) Architectures of trauma: forced shelter and immigration detention. In: Scott-Smith T, Breeze ME (eds) Structures of protection? Rethinking refugee shelter. Berghahn Books, New York

Nematy A, Namer Y, Razum O (2022) LGBTQI+ refugees' and asylum seekers' mental health: a qualitative systematic review. Sex Res Soc Policy 26:636–663

O'Leary CH (2019) Addressing the epidemic of sexual assault in California's immigration detention centres. UCLA Centre for the Study of Women, Policy Brief 25. Available at: https://escholarship.org/content/qt3t0126k9/qt3t0126k9.pdf

Oliveira C, Keygnaert I, Rosário M, Martins O, Dias S (2018) Assessing reported cases of sexual and gender-based violence, causes and preventive strategies, in European asylum reception facilities. Glob Health 14(1):1–12

Passardi S, Hocking DC, Morina N, Sundram S, Alisic E (2022) Moral injury related to immigration detention on Nauru: a qualitative study. Eur J Psychotraumatol 13(1)

Perera S, Pugliese J (2021) Sexual violence and the border: colonial genealogies of US and Australian immigration detention regimes. Soc Leg Stud 30(1):66–79

Peterie M (2018) Deprivation, frustration, and trauma: immigration detention centres as prisons. Refug Surv Q 37(3):279–306

Ramsy M (2021) Beyond the U Visa and carceral feminist "crimmigration": transforming the VAWA self-petition to remedy sexual violence in immigration detention. N.Y.U Rev Law Soc Change 45(1):37

Razum O, Butenop J (2022) Camp setting in the EU, Australia, and their etended border zones. In: Razum O, Dawson A, Eckenwiler L, Wild V (eds) Refugee camps in Europe and Australia: an interdisciplinary critique, pp 47–64

Rivas L, Bull M (2018) Gender and risk: an empirical examination of the experiences of women held in long-term immigration detention in Australia. Refug Surv Q 37(3):307–327

Silverman SJ, Griffiths M, Walsh PW (2022) Immigration detention in the UK'. The Migration Observatory at the University of Oxford. Available at: https://migrationobservatory.ox.ac.uk/resources/briefings/immigration-detention-in-the-uk/

Steinerte E (2022) Liberty of person, right to. In: Binder C, Nowak M, Hofbauer JA, Janig P (eds) Elgar encyclopedia of human rights. Edward Elgar Publishing, Cheltenham

Stirling-Cameron E, Goldenberg S (2022) The detention of migrants in Canadian jails is a public health emergency. The Conversation. Available at: https://theconversation.com/the-detention-of-migrants-in-canadian-jails-is-a-public-health-emergency-194968

Tabak S, Levitan R (2014) LGBTI migrants in immigration detention: a global perspective. Harv J Law Gend 37(1)

Tan SE, Kuschminder K (2022) Migrant experiences of sexual and gender based violence: a critical interpretive synthesis. Glob Health 18:68

Tschalaer M (2023) Queering migration temporalities: LGBTQI+ experiences while waiting within Germany's asylum system. Ethn Racial Stud 46(9):1833–1853

Turnbull S (2017) Immigration detention and punishment. Criminol Crim Just. https://doi.org/10.1093/acrefore/9780190264079.013.231

United Nations High Commissioner for Refugees (UNHCR) (2018) Compilation of international human rights law and standards on immigration detention. Available at: https://www.refworld.org/docid/5afc25c24.html

United Nations Working Group on Arbitrary Detention (2019) Revised Fact Sheet No. 26. Available at: https://www.ohchr.org/sites/default/files/Documents/Issues/Detention/FactSheet26.pdf

United Nations High Commissioner for Refugees (UNHCR) (2020) Global strategy beyond detention 2014–2019: Final progress report. Available at: https://www.refworld.org/pdfid/5f452dce4.pdf

Vasefi S, Dehm S (2022) Refugee women and the gendered violence of Australia's extraterritorial asylum regime on Nauru. Refug Surv Q 41(3):529–558

Weiler G, Bartovic J, Bischoff Ebbesen B, Gottardo C, Puthoopparambil SJ (2022) Improving health in immigration detention and promoting alternatives to detention. Lancet 399(10338):1849–1850

Women's Refugee Commission (2019) "More Than One Million Pains": sexual violence against men and boys on the Central Mediterranean Route to Italy. https://www.womensrefugeecommission.org/research-resources/more-than-one-million-pains-sexual-violence-against-men-and-boys-on-the-central-mediterranean-route-to-italy/

Wood LCN (2018) Impact of punitive immigration policies, parent-child separation and child detention on the mental health and development of children. BMJ Paediatr Open 2:e000338

World Health Organization (2022a) Addressing the health challenges in immigration detention, and alternatives to detention. Available at: https://iris.who.int/handle/10665/353569

World Health Organization (2022b) World report on the health of refugees and migrants. Available at: https://www.who.int/publications/i/item/9789240054462

Caring for Refugees and Migrants: Volunteer and Professional Aid Workers

9

Anne Jachmann and Katharina Wahedi

Contents

The original version of the chapter has been revised. A correction to this chapter can be found at https://doi.org/10.1007/978-3-032-20707-4_12

A. Jachmann (✉)
Department of Emergency Medicine, Inselspital, University Hospital Bern, University of Bern, Bern, Switzerland

Department of Medicine, Swiss Tropical and Public Health Institute, Allschwil, Switzerland

University of Basel, Basel, Switzerland
e-mail: anne.jachmann@insel.ch

K. Wahedi
Department of Emergency Medicine, Inselspital, University Hospital Bern, University of Bern, Bern, Switzerland

Abstract

Volunteer and professional aid workers providing care to migrants and refugees, particularly survivors of sexual violence, frequently endure high levels of stress, demanding and complex work and face an elevated risk of physical and mental distress. It is therefore crucial to provide access to tailored, needs-based training and mental health support services that equip aid workers with the skills,

V. Padovese, I. Rossoni (eds.), *Intersections of Sexual Health, Migration and Sexualised Violence*, Sustainable Development Goals Series, https://doi.org/10.1007/978-3-032-20707-4_9

knowledge, and awareness necessary to address these challenges effectively. These measures not only reduce stress but also enhance professional competence and resilience, enable identification of and response to mental and physical health risks, and help maintain empathy and motivation in challenging circumstances.

Beyond improving overall health, the continuous acquisition, maintenance, and expansion of professional expertise among refugee aid workers contribute to the provision of high-quality care. Well-trained and adequately supported workers are better prepared to address the diverse needs of those they serve and to deliver compassionate, effective, and competent care to refugees and migrants. This chapter outlines the individual and systemic factors required to promote the provision of appropriate services in humanitarian settings and to strengthen the well-being of aid workers.

Keywords

Refugee aid worker · Humanitarian aid · Competencies · Mental health · Stress relief · Resilience · Training

9.1 Introduction

Migration has always been a fundamental part of human existence; throughout history, people have moved and changed their place of living, either voluntarily in search of better opportunities or forced to do so in search of safety or survival. The contemporary migration experience is often characterized by significant changes in living conditions, challenges and experiences of violence and insecurity along the journey, and precarious circumstances that can have a profound impact on the lives and health of migrants and refugees. It is therefore not surprising that migration is often seen as a key determinant of health.

Any volunteer or professional caring for refugees and migrants, regardless of their discipline or work setting, is confronted with these challenges and experiences faced by refugees and migrants. Yet, the training of aid workers often fails to adequately prepare them to provide holistic care and to identify, assess, and address the complex obstacles that these individuals face during life-changing events, such as displacement and resettlement.

Aid work in general is inherently demanding and emotionally exhausting, requiring aid workers to navigate the suffering of migrants and refugees, manage complex situations, conflicts, and multiple needs, and make time-sensitive decisions on a daily basis (Jachmann and Karamagioli 2021). Adding to the strain, refugee aid workers (RAWs) often operate in unstable, harsh environments, where institutional barriers, financial constraints, and scarce resources severely hinder the ability to provide effective, high-quality care (Jachmann et al. 2024).

RAWs in migration and health face complex contextual challenges, such as political and sociocultural factors, alongside the limits of (medical) care action and pressure to act beyond their professional expertise and capacity, often leading to overextension, ethical dilemmas, disillusionment, and exposure to injustice (Jachmann et al. 2024). Working in the field of sexual and reproductive health adds another layer of complexity, as RAWs are frequently exposed to violations of sexual and reproductive rights. The impact of witnessing such violations, combined with the challenging political, religious, and socio-cultural structures in which RAWs operate, exacerbates the difficulties of providing adequate care and support.

At the same time, these violations and challenges can give rise to personal struggles for RAWs, which may become particularly difficult to navigate when viewed as an individual failing, personal responsibility, or fault. This is further compounded when such struggles are suppressed out of a belief that they should not exist in the first place.

This chapter shows that such problems are often systemic and collective, rather than isolated. They require solutions that address the underlying systemic factors to ensure a more comprehensive and effective response.

Understanding both the positive and negative impacts of working in these contexts is essential to identifying and assessing individual struggles. However, the tools and frameworks to address these challenges are often not well known or readily available. This chapter aims to provide resources, strategies, and insights needed to understand and effectively address the challenges of working in such contexts.

9.2 Impact of Migration and Refugee Health (MRH) Work

9.2.1 Impact on Private Life

Working in the field of migration and health can have both positive and negative effects on the aid worker and their environment, depending on the attitudes of those around them. Amid the rise of political nationalism, anti-migration movements, and the increasing politicization of migration, staff working with migrants and refugees may encounter social stigmatization or feel reluctant to discuss their work. This can contribute to tensions or social divisions within families, neighborhoods, and communities. On the other hand, positive attitudes from those around them can also lead to recognition, support and appreciation.

Working abroad during missions can cause separation from family and children leading to feelings of loss, breakups, or divorce (Robinson 2002). Interruptions in intimate relationships can be caused by longer distance while being away on missions abroad or by vicarious trauma (Rizkalla and Segal 2020). Furthermore, aid workers who support survivors of sexual violence may experience secondary traumatic stress (STS) associated with a decline in sexual intimacy, as well as shifts in maintaining closeness and their ability to trust others (Rizkalla and Segal 2019).

9.2.2 Impact on Mental Health

Professionals and volunteers working in migration and refugee health are routinely exposed to extreme stress and psychological strain, often resulting in the emergence or aggravation of emotional disorders such as burnout, post-traumatic stress disorder (PTSD), anxiety, or depression (Jachmann et al. 2024). These conditions can severely compromise their performance, leading to shifts in behavior, such as diminished empathy or patience and to a heightened risk of medical errors that can undermine the quality of care and treatment outcomes for refugees and migrants (Jachmann et al. 2024; Williams et al. 2007; Wallace et al. 2009; Motowidlo et al. 1986). RAWs are often exposed to the trauma of others, which can lead to secondary traumatic stress (STS) or secondary traumatization and can manifest in symptoms similar to those of PTSD, such as emotional exhaustion, anxiety, depression, disturbed sleep patterns, and emotional numbing (Figley 1995). This has been shown in various distinct settings, including medical students working a few hours a week in an outpatient clinic at a reception center in Germany (Kindermann et al. 2019) and translators working in an ambulatory clinic (Kindermann et al. 2017). Furthermore, the risk of developing PTSD, depression, and anxiety was found to be heightened by exposure to trauma, with the severity of depressive symptoms linked to the number of traumatic events experienced (Eriksson et al. 2013; Borho et al. 2019). Building on previous reviews of the literature (Jachmann et al. 2024), studies on RAWs reveal high rates of psychological conditions (Eriksson et al. 2013; Borho et al. 2019; Chatzea et al. 2018; Espinosa et al. 2019; Brooks et al. 2022; Živanović and Vukčević Marković 2020; Suzic et al. 2016; Chemali et al. 2017; Roberts et al. 2021), including anxiety (20–50.4%), burnout (29.7–57%), PTSD (3.6–44.7%), psychological distress (36.5%), and depression (10.1–55.2%). With regard to symptoms of STS, these were shown in 22.9–51.3% of RAWs (Espinosa et al. 2019; Brooks et al. 2022; Živanović and Vukčević Marković 2020; Suzic et al. 2016; Roberts et al. 2021; Denkinger et al. 2018; Kim 2017) and for vicarious trauma in 26% (Rizkalla and Segal 2020; Mishori et al. 2014).

Additionally, when professionals listen to refugee's recount experiences of pain, fear, and suffering, they may begin to feel similar emotions due to their deep empathy and concern (Rizkalla and Segal 2020; Figley 1995). This can sometimes blur their sense of self, merging it with the experiences of those they serve, especially when the professional shares the same cultural history or experiences (Splevins et al. 2010). For example, therapists working with survivors of sexual assault might develop a broader sense of aversion toward men, while those supporting victims of different crimes may start feeling heightened fears for their own safety, leading them to seek additional security measures (Figley 1995; Iliffe and Steed 2000). RAWs may also experience moral distress when they are unable to provide the care or services they believe are necessary due to systemic limitations. This can create a conflict between personal values and professional responsibilities, contributing to stress and dissatisfaction, as was shown in a study of moral distress among nurses working in resource-constrained settings during the COVID-19 pandemic (Gustavsson et al. 2023).

Despite all the challenges, there are countless positive aspects to working in this context. Many RAWs reported that their experiences working with refugees have profoundly and positively transformed their lives, leading to shifts in their life philosophy, deeper self-awareness, and enriched interpersonal relationships, where intentional efforts to find meaning in their work contributed to the positive transformation (Barrington and Shakespeare-Finch 2013). In addition, a reduction in the risk of depression and anxiety was linked to a prolonged career in the humanitarian sector (Eriksson et al. 2013).

9.2.3 Impact on Physical Health

High levels of stress can increase the occurrence of cardiovascular risk factors and complications such as acute myocardial infarction or even sudden cardiac death, especially when low job control is combined with high demand or effort (Siegrist 1996; Jachmann et al. 2024; Kivimäki et al. 2002). Studies have shown that other causes of death during field missions, mainly in Africa, were riots or other acts of violence, accidents, or infections, while evacuations during fieldwork were mainly due to infectious diseases, accidents, obstetric-gynecological conditions, or preexisting medical problems (e.g., cancer) (Peytremann et al. 2006; Schouten and Borgdorff 1995; Lange et al. 2006). More comprehensive use of standard preventive measures, such as safe food and water practices, malaria prophylaxis, mosquito avoidance strategies, and adequate immunizations, could have helped prevent or lessen some cases of morbidity as well as predeparture medical checks (Lange et al. 2006). Working in the field can also expose RAWs to dangerous conditions, where their personal security and health is at high risk, such as explosions, kidnapping, attacks, different types of violence and torture, or climate-related hazards (Staff UNHCR 2020). Moreover, rising levels of STS and a reduced connection to the organization seem to be both linked to worsened physical health (Rizkalla and Segal 2019).

9.2.4 Impact on the System

The high psychological and physical burden of demanding aid work can lead to loss of productivity, including through sick leave. Other consequences include high staff turnover and leaving the humanitarian sector or leaving the profession altogether (e.g. medicine) (Chemali et al. 2017; Jachmann et al. 2024; Coffa 2016). The high cost of recruiting and training new staff puts further pressure on an already overstretched system. In addition, high turnover rates also have a negative impact on the collective experience of the team (Fig. 9.1).

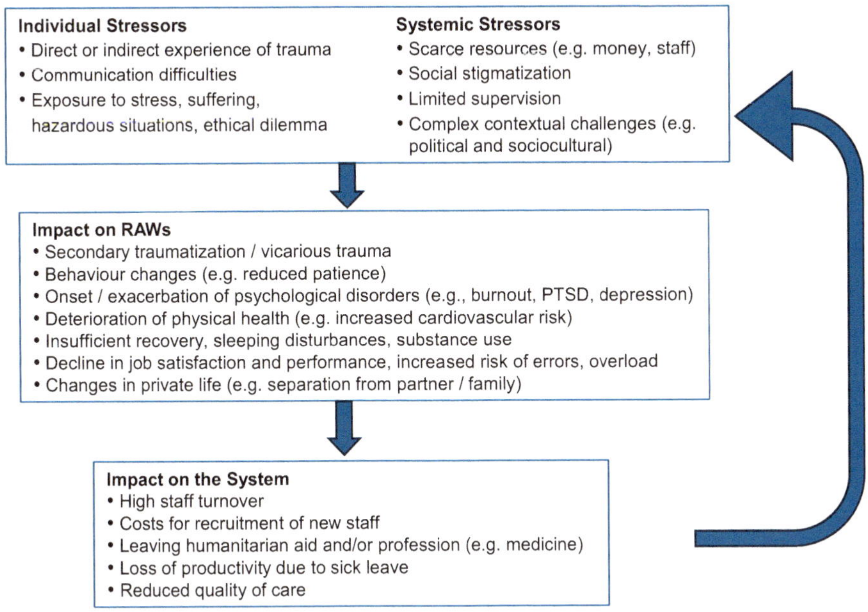

Fig. 9.1 Working in the field of MRH: exposure to stressors and their potential negative impacts. Adapted from Jachmann et al. 2024

9.3 Required Core Competencies in the Field of MRH

9.3.1 Guidelines, Frameworks, and Operational Models for Care Providers

Migrants and refugees are often exposed to multiple social, psychological, and legal risk factors which can create significant barriers to accessing healthcare. These challenges include an uncertain residence status, lack of work permit, living in asylum centers or overcrowded housing, and language barriers.

When providing (health) care, it is therefore essential to consider and address the diverse social determinants of health and complex circumstances faced by individuals who have migrated. The biopsychosocial model, introduced by George Engel (1977), is an approach to healthcare that emphasizes the interaction between biological, psychological, and social factors that influence health, enabling (health) care professionals to follow a holistic approach.

Applying the biopsychosocial model when assessing the health status and needs of individuals with a migration background is crucial, as it allows for a comprehensive understanding of how social determinants of health impact these individuals. This approach calls for specialized training for (health) care professionals, strong interprofessional collaboration, and the creation of a well-connected network of (health) care providers who work together in close coordination (Jachmann et al. 2025; Cignacco et al. 2018).

Smooth teamwork, clear and understandable communication, and a supportive environment are key to effectively addressing the complex needs of migrants and refugees.

It is therefore highly recommended that organizations providing humanitarian services in the area of MRH identify the key stakeholders active in their setting and establish a network for collaboration. This, together with exploring models of good practice and established frameworks, will enable organizations to effectively structure and improve their services to address the challenges outlined above with greater impact. Crucially, this entails adapting health information, promotion and prevention strategies, and other provided services to the specific needs and vulnerabilities of the respective target populations (Jachmann et al. 2022).

In response to the demand for quality assurance and professionalism in the humanitarian sector, various guidelines, frameworks, and operational models have been developed. These models include competency standards, which outline the essential skills and knowledge required for (health) care providers working in the field of MRH. The standards, as described by WHO (World Health Organization 2021) in figure 9.2, are intended to ensure that professionals in the field are equipped to meet the challenges of providing care to these vulnerable populations (Fig. 9.2).

Similar frameworks exist for the context of sexual and reproductive health (SRH). For example, the WHO «framework for ensuring human rights in the provision of contraceptive information and services» (World Health Organization 2014) applies a human rights approach to the delivery of these services. With regard to the provision of SRH services and information, the framework highlights the following key dimensions: acceptability, non-discrimination, accessibility, availability, quality, accountability,

Competency Standards in refugee and migrant health as listed by WHO	Domain
• Provision of people-centered (health) care • Fostering refugees' and migrants' agency and empowerment at all levels (individual & community)	*People-centeredness*
• Addressing communication & language needs with safe and appropriate measures • Ensuring refugees and migrants understanding of their (health) care information	*Communication*
• Promoting the health of refugees and migrants through collaborative practice • Responding to increased service demand related to migration and displacement	*Collaboration*
• Advancing refugee`s and migrant`s evidence-informed (health) care	*Evidence-informed practice*
• Promoting the health of refugees and migrants through engagement in reflective practice and lifelong learning • Contributing to a culture of mutual support and self-care	*Personal conduct*

Fig. 9.2 Required core competencies in the field of MRH according to the World Health Organization (WHO) Global Competency Standards for health workers providing services to refugees and migrants (World Health Organization 2021)

informed-decision-making, participation, confidentiality, and privacy (World Health Organization 2014).

The International Organization for Migration (IOM) has also established an «Institutional Framework for Addressing Gender-Based Violence in Crisis» (International Organization for Migration (IOM) 2018). This framework focuses on three core areas: (1) mitigating risks of gender-based violence during crisis operations to prevent harm, (2) supporting survivors by improving access to services, and (3) addressing the underlying causes that enable gender-based violence. Another framework developed by the Global Health and Protection Cluster (Global Health Cluster, Global Protection Cluster 2023) emphasizes the importance of adequate coordination of both health and protection responses during crisis. It also provides good practice examples and guidance on how to connect health and protection actors, to promote cross-sectoral collaboration and entails templates for referral forms and checklists for health services accessibility and availability.

9.4 Strengthening Refugee Aid Worker: Protective Factors and Supportive Measures

9.4.1 Individual Protective and Risk Factors

The perception of emotions and the impact of personal experiences on overall well-being depend on numerous factors, including professional training and expertise, individual characteristics, such as personality traits, and life experiences (Lu et al. 2014). Personality traits, such as hardiness, optimism, and self-efficacy play a crucial role in mitigating post-traumatic risk of developing vicarious trauma (Sifaki-Pistolla et al. 2017). People with high self-efficacy believe they can influence events in their lives and effectively manage difficult situations (Bandura 1982). Research on rescue workers indicates that self-efficacy is strongly linked with reduced mental health distress, such as fewer symptoms of traumatic stress or depression (Chatzea et al. 2018; Heinrichs et al. 2005; Mao et al. 2022). Hardiness is a related concept that encompasses self-efficacy while adding two additional dimensions: a deep commitment to one's life activities and the perception of change as an exciting opportunity for personal growth (Kobasa 1979). Together, these traits help individuals navigate adversity more effectively, enhancing resilience in high-stress environments. Considering this and the high stress levels inherent in humanitarian work, particularly in MRH, self-efficacy and hardiness might be crucial in determining an individual's ability to cope with these challenges. Social support from the community has also been shown to be a strong protective factor from developing secondary traumatization (Setti and Argentero 2016; Boscarino et al. 2004).

The stigma associated with being perceived as «not resilient enough» or «weak», and the belief that their own struggles are insignificant compared to those of the people they care for, often prevent RAWs from accepting or seeking support, possibly leading to unwholesome coping strategies, such as enhanced intake of caffeine, nicotine, or other substances (Rizkalla and Segal 2020; Jachmann et al. 2024; Stevens et al. 2022; Dunkley 2018). However, it is important to acknowledge that the constant stress typical in refugee aid work frequently impacts their health. A good stress response is therefore essential. Stress management is not an innate trait but a skill that can be developed over time enabling a person to better navigate recurring stressors and to recognize signs of excessive stress and early warning signals of mental health distress. These and other practices are crucial and non-negotiable aspects of the job, like open communication, regular sharing, self-care, continuous education, and adequate support of mental well-being (Jachmann et al. 2024; Barrington and Shakespeare-Finch 2013). Just as a professional diver would never dive without maintaining their gear properly and performing a thorough equipment check, RAWs who consistently engage in stress reduction, education, training, and self-care practices are better equipped to stay focused, robust, empathetic, engaged, and resilient in the face of challenges (Jachmann et al. 2024).

Effective, well-established strategies for enhancing well-being and stress management include (Rizkalla and Segal 2020; Jachmann et al. 2024; Dunkley 2018) ensuring regular physical activity and restful sleep; maintaining a healthy and balanced diet; avoiding excessive or unhealthy consumption of substances (e.g., cigarettes, alcohol) or internet use; practicing self-care; incorporating daily relaxation routines, such as engaging in hobbies, meditation, or yoga; maintaining regular communication with friends, family, or colleagues; planning for recovery periods (e.g., taking vacations or breaks between assignments); and reducing work-related stress by sharing tasks and managing workload.

9.4.2 Systemic Protective and Risk Factors

Besides the described individual factors, systemic protective factors also play a crucial role in managing stress and the risk for mental health or post-traumatic distress. A study among 782 rescue workers identified role clarity and job support as important factors influencing vicarious traumatization (Argentero and Setti 2011). Role clarity was considered the degree of clarity with regard to allocated duties and responsibility and job support as the support of co-workers and superiors (Argentero and Setti 2011).

Similarly, other studies with RAWs have identified social support/team cohesion as key protective (resilience) factors against anxiety/burnout (Eriksson et al. 2013) and have shown that feeling connected to the organization (NGO) can be considered a protective factor, as poorer physical health and well-being are associated with less connection to the organization (Rizkalla and Segal 2019). Trust in the team management alleviated the negative effects of working in a high autonomy context in a study with expatriates of Medecins Sans Frontieres (Visser et al. 2016).

On the other hand, factors contributing to vicarious trauma include limited resources, worries about personal safety, insufficient benefits, lack of adequate equipment, challenging living conditions, high caseloads, demanding organizational expectations, and exposure to trauma narratives (Rizkalla and Segal 2020). Additionally, providers are at higher risk of developing STS due to frequent interactions with trauma clients, a personal history of trauma, limited experience, overcommitment, effort-reward imbalance, or heavy caseloads (Rizkalla and Segal 2019; Suzic et al. 2016). An imbalance between effort and reward has been identified as a strong predictor of increased risk for depression, PTSD, and Burnout in RAWs (Suzic et al. 2016).

Raising awareness of mental health distress and providing professional psychological support within organizations and the humanitarian sector in general are crucial and can be achieved by educational campaigns on conditions such as PTSD to help RAWs recognize early signs of distress and create a more open environment for discussion and treatment (Sifaki-Pistolla et al. 2017). Awareness-raising initiatives are particularly important for RAWs at the start of their careers, as knowledge of distress and coping strategies is often limited, and less time spent in the field is associated with a higher risk of mental distress, such as anxiety or depression (Eriksson et al. 2013). Supervision is also essential, not only for inexperienced aid workers but for everyone involved in the field of MRH, with studies quantifying this need at 61–72% (Rizkalla and Segal 2020; Eriksson et al. 2013; Denkinger et al. 2018; Splevins et al. 2010). This is particularly relevant when working with individuals who have experienced violence or torture. Organizations need to ensure that their staff are adequately trained and supervised and that a supportive, cohesive working environment is fostered to help them meet the demands of their roles (Rizkalla and Segal 2020; Barrington and Shakespeare-Finch 2013). Optimizing work organization is another critical factor in safeguarding the mental health of employees, which can include implementing shorter shifts, creating efficient rotation schedules, and ensuring ample rest periods to promote well-being (Sifaki-Pistolla et al. 2017).

9.4.3 Preparation and Support Measures for RAWs

Adequate preparation of RAWs should ideally be preceded by screening for preexisting psychological distress and identification of individuals who already practice appropriate coping strategies and are resilient (Sifaki-Pistolla et al. 2017; Lopes Cardozo et al. 2012). This should be followed by a detailed briefing on the procedures, content, and potential consequences of the intended job assignment, including distress and STS preventive measures, a risk analysis and disaster preparedness training. Ideally additional briefings take place during and after the deployment, combined with assessments to identify needs for support.

Continuous training and further education to foster professional development and expertise is indispensable as it equips RAWs with the necessary skills and knowledge to provide adequate services. In addition, organizations should regularly train teams together to ensure they are adequately prepared (including rescue and disaster preparedness, such as an outbreak of fire or infectious disease), to promote smooth operations, and to reduce adverse incidents, distress and the risk of exposure to infection, trauma, or hazards (Chatzea et al. 2018).

In addition to regular training, other support services, such as mental health care, should be available and accessible at all times, regardless of where and at what stage a RAW is before, during, and after deployment. Well-trained and adequately supported workers are better prepared to address the diverse needs of those they serve and to deliver compassionate, effective, and competent care to refugees and migrants (Fig. 9.3).

9.5 Tools & Courses for Advanced Training and Skills Acquisition

9.5.1 Training for Professionals Working within MRH

- Free online courses from WHO experts in more than 60 national and local languages: https://whoacademy.org/coursewares?search=migration
- Yearly hybrid WHO Global School on Refugee and Migrant Health: https://www.who.int/news-room/events/detail/2024/12/02/default-calendar/fifth-who-global-school-on-refugee-and-migrant-health
- Training and capacity building programs on migration and health by IOM for health professionals, social workers, immigration officers or other border officials: https://eea.iom.int/training-migration-and-health
- A virtual course for health professionals on MRH available in 24 languages, established by the consortium "Train 4 Migrant & Health" and property of the European Commission: https://learning.ecdc.europa.eu/totara/catalog/explore.php?catalog_fts=migration%20and%20health
- Paloma Training consists of training material and a guidebook for the care and counselling of refugees (e.g., working with an interpreter) by the Finnish Institute for Health and Welfare (THL): https://thl.fi/en/topics/migration-and-cultural-diversity/support-material/paloma-training
- Online course on anti-racism for professionals by the Finnish Institute for Health and Welfare (THL): https://thl.fi/en/topics/migration-and-cultural-diversity/support-material/online-course-on-anti-racism-for-professionals
- Hands on training programs for professionals working in the field of MRH in Switzerland and globally by the department of emergency

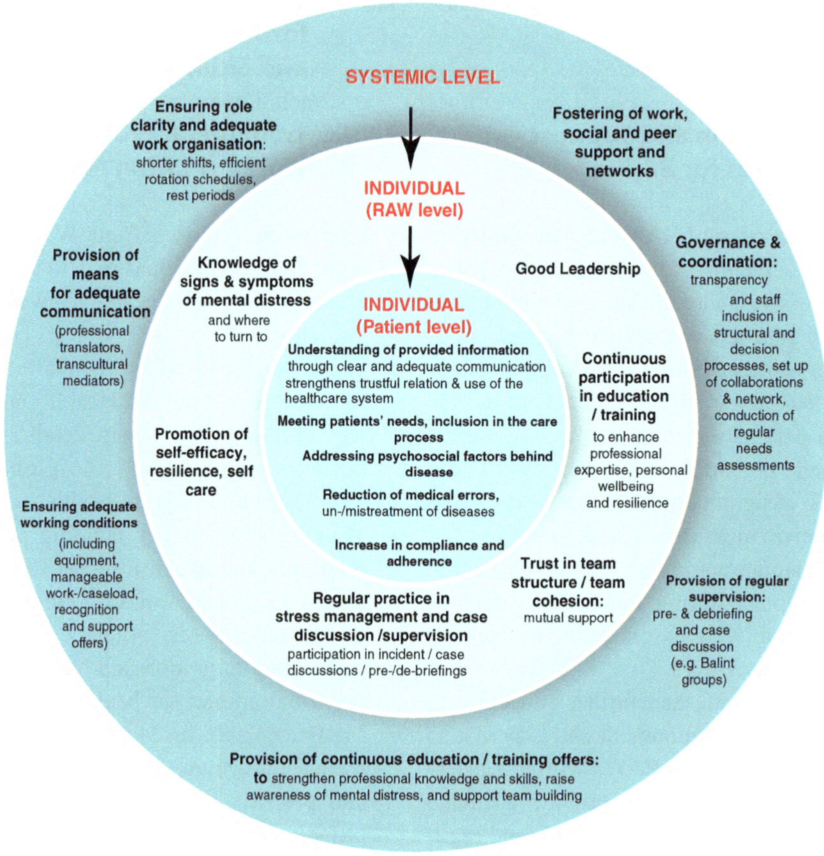

Fig. 9.3 Protective factors and their consequences within MRH work. Adapted from Jachmann et al. 2024 and Jachmann et al. 2025

medicine, Bern University hospital (Inselspital), University of Bern, Switzerland: www.migration-health.com
- Online open course on migration, health, and equity in Europe for professionals working in the public health, policy, education, or research sector, as well as for health professionals by the Geneva Centre of Humanitarian Studies: https://www.unige.ch/medecine/humanitarianstudies/education/our-courses/migration-health-equity-europe

9.5.2 Training Material in the Field of Sexual Health, Migration, and Sexualized Violence

- «Triage Tool for identification, care and referral of victims of sexual violence at European asylum reception and accommodation initiatives» by Keygnaert, I. & Linthout, L. (2020), Ghent University, Ghent. ISBN: 9789078128632: https://biblio.ugent.be/publication/8700886

- «Sexual and Reproductive Health Care In Emergencies» toolkit by the FP2030, an international network: https://www.fp2030.org/resources/ready-to-save-lives-sexual-and-reproductive-health-care-in-emergencies-toolkit/
- Guide by UNHCR for implementation of high quality and life-saving sexual and reproductive health services in humanitarian settings: https://emergency.unhcr.org/emergency-assistance/health-and-nutrition/sexual-and-reproductive-health-including-hiv#3

9.5.3 Training Material for Stress Management

- Guidelines and training offerss for stress management on different levels (individual/responder, team leader, and organizational/agency) for the humanitarian aid and emergency response sector by the Antares Foundation: http://www.antaresfoundation.org
- Collection of resources for stress management, burnout, resilience, staff care, mental health, ethic,s and organizational culture in the humanitarian aid sector by the International Association of Professionals in Humanitarian Assistance and Protection: https://phap.org/PHAP/Sector_Monitoring/Themes/Personal_effectiveness/Health_wellbeing/PHAP/Themes/Health%20and%20wellbeing.aspx
- Information on stress and how to manage it by the U.S. Centers for Disease Control and prevention (CDC): https://www.cdc.gov/mental-health/living-with/index.html
- Guide «Doing What Matters in Times of Stress» by WHO for stress management with audio exercises to cope with adversity. Available in 33 languages (ISBN: 9789240003927): https://www.who.int/publications/i/item/9789240003927?gclid=CjwKCAjwqJSaBhBUEiwAg5W9pz0tHY4I_Wf8kd4SWs147UR0mTSWLil3YwV89eRtVM74gZb3pnlzZxoCWU0QAvD_BwE
- Resource portal for disaster and first responders, including online training for stress management, preparation for deployment, peer support by the Disaster Technical Assistance Center (DTAC) of the Substance Abuse and Mental Health Services Administration (SAMHSA): https://www.samhsa.gov/dtac/disaster-responders

Acknowledgments The AI large language models (LLMs) of ChatGPT (OpenAI 2024) and Deepl Write (DeepL 2024) were used to improve readability and language of this chapter.

References

Argentero P, Setti I (2011) Engagement and vicarious traumatization in rescue workers. Int Arch Occup Environ Health 84(1):67–75

Bandura A (1982) Self-efficacy mechanism in human agency. Am Psychol 37(2):122–147

Barrington AJ, Shakespeare-Finch J (2013) Working with refugee survivors of torture and trauma: an opportunity for vicarious post-traumatic growth. Couns Psychol Q 26(1):89–105

Borho A, Georgiadou E, Grimm T, Morawa E, Silbermann A, Nißlbeck W et al (2019) Professional and volunteer refugee aid workers–depressive symptoms and their predictors, experienced traumatic events, PTSD, burdens, engagement motivators and support needs. Int J Environ Res Public Health 16(22):4542

Boscarino JA, Figley CR, Adams RE (2004) Compassion fatigue following the September 11 terrorist attacks: a study of secondary trauma among New York City social workers. Int J Emerg Ment Health 6(2):57–66

Brooks MA, Dasgupta A, Taşğın NŞ, Meinhart M, Tekin U, Yükseker D et al (2022) Secondary traumatic stress, depression, and anxiety symptoms among service providers working with Syrian refugees in Istanbul, Turkey. J Immigr Minor Health 24(6):1421–1430

Chatzea VE, Sifaki-Pistolla D, Vlachaki SA, Melidoniotis E, Pistolla G (2018) PTSD, burnout and well-being among rescue workers: seeking to understand the impact of the European refugee crisis on rescuers. Psychiatry Res 262:446–451

Chemali Z, Borba CPC, Johnson K, Hock RS, Parnarouskis L, Henderson DC et al (2017) Humanitarian space and well-being: effectiveness of training on a psychosocial intervention for host community-refugee interaction. Med Confl Surviv 33(2):141–161

Cignacco E, zu Sayn-Wittgenstein F, Sénac C, Hurni A, Wyssmüller D, Grand-Guillaume-Perrenoud JA et al (2018) Sexual and reproductive healthcare for women asylum seekers in Switzerland: a multi-method evaluation. BMC Health Serv Res 18(1):712

Coffa D (2016) Caring for ourselves while caring for others. In: King TE, Wheeler MB (eds) Medical management of vulnerable and underserved patients: principles, practice, and populations, 2e. McGraw-Hill Education, New York

DeepL (2024) DeepL Write, Free Online Version, DeepL SE in Cologne, Germany. https://www.deepl.com/write

Denkinger JK, Windthorst P, Rometsch-Ogioun El Sount C, Blume M, Sedik H, Kizilhan JI et al (2018) Secondary traumatization in caregivers working with women and children who suffered extreme violence by the "Islamic State". Front Psychiatry 9:234

Dunkley F (2018) 1. Introduction & 4. Resilience toolkit. In: Psychosocial support for humanitarian aid workers: a roadmap of trauma and critical incident care, 1st edn. Routledge

Engel GL (1977) The need for a new medical model: a challenge for biomedicine. Science 196(4286):129–136

Eriksson CB, Lopes Cardozo B, Ghitis F, Sabin M, Gotway Crawford C, Zhu J et al (2013) Factors associated with adverse mental health outcomes in locally recruited aid workers assisting Iraqi refugees in Jordan. J Aggress Maltreat Trauma 22(6):660–680

Espinosa A, Akinsulure-Smith AM, Chu T (2019) Trait emotional intelligence, coping, and occupational distress among resettlement workers. Psychol Trauma Theory Res Pract Policy 11:28–34

Figley CR (1995) Compassion fatigue as secondary traumatic stress disorder: an overview. In: Figley CR (ed) Compassion fatigue: coping with secondary traumatic stress disorder in those who treat the traumatized, 1st edn. Routledge, pp 1–20

Global Health Cluster, Global Protection Cluster (2023) Joint Operational Framework Health and Protection. Global Health Cluster, Global Protection Cluster, editors. Geneva, 37 p

Gustavsson ME, von Schreeb J, Arnberg FK, Juth N (2023) Being prevented from providing good care: a conceptual analysis of moral stress among health care workers during the COVID-19 pandemic. BMC Med Ethics 24(1):110

Heinrichs M, Wagner D, Schoch W, Soravia LM, Hellhammer DH, Ehlert U (2005) Predicting posttraumatic stress symptoms from pretraumatic risk factors: a 2-year prospective follow-up study in firefighters. Am J Psychiatry 162(12):2276–2286

Iliffe G, Steed LG (2000) Exploring the counselor's experience of working with perpetrators and survivors of domestic violence. J Interpers Violence 15(4):393–412

International Organization for Migration (IOM) (2018) Department of Operations and Emergencies (DOE). Institutional framework for addressing gender-based violence in crisis. Geneva, 40 p

Jachmann A, Karamagioli E (2021) Round table: Strengthening refugee aid workers resilience during the pandemic and beyond. Eur J Public Health 31(3):6. ckab164.469, https://doi.org/10.1093/eurpub/ckab164.469

Jachmann A, Saffuri R, Eijer H, Brown AD, Karamagioli E, et al. (2022) Trauma consultations in a Swiss tertiary emergency department: Comparison of asylum seekers and the local population — Patient characteristics and patterns of injuries, a retrospective study. PLOS ONE 17(11): e0277418. https://doi.org/10.1371/journal.pone.0277418

Jachmann A, Exadaktylos A, Paris D (2024) Tätigkeit im Bereich Migration und Gesundheit: Herausforderungen, Auswirkungen und Empfehlungen. In: Exadaktylos A, Keidar O, Srivastava DS, Paris DH (eds) Migrations-und Flüchtlingsmedizin: Ein Praxisleitfaden für die Primär- und Grundversorgung. Hogrefe AG, Bern, pp 67–74

Jachmann A, Brandenberger J, Schick M (2025) Equitable health care in the context of migration. Swiss Med Wkly [Internet] 155(3):4245. https://doi.org/10.57187/s.4245

Kim YJ (2017) Secondary traumatic stress and burnout of North Korean refugees service providers. Psychiatry Investig 14(2):118–125

Kindermann D, Schmid C, Derreza-Greeven C, Huhn D, Kohl RM, Junne F et al (2017) Prevalence of and risk factors for secondary traumatization in interpreters for refugees: a cross-sectional study. Psychopathology 50(4):262–272

Kindermann D, Jenne MP, Schmid C, Bozorgmehr K, Wahedi K, Junne F et al (2019) Motives, experiences and psychological strain in medical students engaged in refugee care in a reception center– a mixed-methods approach. BMC Med Educ 19(1):302

Kivimäki M, Leino-Arjas P, Luukkonen R, Riihimäki H, Vahtera J, Kirjonen J (2002) Work stress and risk of cardiovascular mortality: prospective cohort study of industrial employees. BMJ 325(7369):857

Kobasa SC (1979) Stressful life events, personality, and health: an inquiry into hardiness. J Pers Soc Psychol 37(1):1–11

Lange WR, Frankenfield DL, Frame JD (2006) Morbidity among refugee relief workers. J Travel Med 1(2):111–112

Lopes Cardozo B, Gotway Crawford C, Eriksson C, Zhu J, Sabin M, Ager A et al (2012) Psychological distress, depression, anxiety, and burnout among international humanitarian aid workers: a longitudinal study. PLoS One 7(9):e44948

Lu J, Yang N, Ye J, Wu H (2014) The influence paths of emotion on the occupational safety of rescuers involved in environmental emergencies- systematic review article. Iran J Public Health 43(11):1478–1485

Mao X, Hu X, Loke AY (2022) A concept analysis on disaster resilience in rescue workers: the psychological perspective. Disaster Med Public Health Prep 16(4):1682–1691

Mishori R, Mujawar I, Ravi N (2014) Self-reported vicarious trauma in asylum evaluators: a preliminary survey. J Immigr Minor Health 16(6):1232–1237
Motowidlo SJ, Packard JS, Manning MR (1986) Occupational stress: its causes and consequences for job performance. J Appl Psychol 71:618–629
OpenAI (2024) ChatGPT (GPT-4), Dezember 2024 Version. OpenAI, https://chat.openai.com
Peytremann I, Baduraux M, O'Donovan S, Loutan L (2006) Medical evacuations and fatalities of United Nations high commissioner for refugees field employees. J Travel Med 8(3):117–121
Rizkalla N, Segal SP (2019) Trauma during humanitarian work: the effects on intimacy, wellbeing and PTSD-symptoms. Eur J Psychotraumatol 10(1):1679065
Rizkalla N, Segal SP (2020) Refugee trauma work: effects on intimate relationships and vicarious posttraumatic growth. J Affect Disord 276:839–847
Roberts F, Teague B, Lee J, Rushworth I (2021) The prevalence of burnout and secondary traumatic stress in professionals and volunteers working with forcibly displaced people: a systematic review and two meta-analyses. J Trauma Stress 34(4):773–785
Robinson K (2002) Voices: separation from families. In: Danieli Y (ed) Sharing the front line and the Back Hills: international protectors and providers: peacekeepers, humanitarian aid workers and the media in the midst of crisis. Routledge, pp 134–135
Schouten EJ, Borgdorff MW (1995) Increased mortality among Dutch development workers. BMJ 311(7016):1343–1344
Setti I, Argentero P (2016) Traumatization and PTSD in rescue workers: prevention, assessment, and interventions. In: Martin CR, Preedy VR, Patel VB (eds) Comprehensive guide to post-traumatic stress disorders. Springer International Publishing, Cham, pp 301–317
Siegrist J (1996) Adverse health effects of high-effort/low-reward conditions. J Occup Health Psychol 1(1):27–41
Sifaki-Pistolla D, Chatzea VE, Vlachaki SA, Melidoniotis E, Pistolla G (2017) Who is going to rescue the rescuers? Post-traumatic stress disorder among rescue workers operating in Greece during the European refugee crisis. Soc Psychiatry Psychiatr Epidemiol 52(1):45–54
Splevins KA, Cohen K, Joseph S, Murray C, Bowley J (2010) Vicarious posttraumatic growth among interpreters. Qual Health Res 20(12):1705–1716
UNHCR Staff (2020) UNHCR chief praises aid workers battling multiple crises: On World Humanitarian Day, Filippo Grandi honours the 'depth of commitment' to a role made 'significantly harder' by COVID-19 [Internet]. United Nations High Commissioner for Refugees (UNHCR); 2020 Aug 19 [cited 2026 Mar 16]. Available from: https://www.unhcr.org/news/stories/unhcr-chief-praises-aid-workers-battling-multiple-crises
Stevens GJ, Sharma A, Skeoch K (2022) Help-seeking attitudes and behaviours among humanitarian aid workers. J Int Humanit Action 7(1):16
Suzic D, Roslyn T, Jachens L, Mihalca L (2016) Staff well-being and mental health in UNHCR. Wairoa Z, Brossard-Salazar C (eds). United Nations High Commissioner for Refugees (UNHCR), Geneva, p 130
Visser M, Mills M, Heyse L, Wittek R, Bollettino V (2016) Work–Life Balance Among Humanitarian Aid Workers. Nonprofit Volunt Sect Q 45(6):1191–1213
Wallace JE, Lemaire JB, Ghali WA (2009) Physician wellness: a missing quality indicator. Lancet 374(9702):1714–1721
Williams ES, Manwell LB, Konrad TR, Linzer M (2007) The relationship of organizational culture, stress, satisfaction, and burnout with physician-reported error and suboptimal patient care: results from the MEMO study. Health Care Manag Rev 32(3):203–212
World Health Organization (2014) Framework for ensuring human rights in the provision of contraceptive information and services. ISBN 978924 1507745, Geneva
World Health Organization (2021) Refugee and migrant health: global competency standards for health workers, Geneva, Licence: CC BY-NC-SA 3.0 IGO, ISBN 978-92-4-003063-3
Živanović M, Vukčević Marković M (2020) Latent structure of secondary traumatic stress, its precursors, and effects on people working with refugees. PLoS One 15(10):e0241545

10 Reaching Out to Those Left Behind: Deployment of Point-of-Care (POC) Testing for Sexually Transmitted Infections (STIs), Including HIV, in Migrant Populations

Valeska Padovese and Karel Blondeel

Contents

Abstract

This chapter will explore the deployment of point-of-care (POC) testing for sexually transmitted infections (STIs) in migrant populations. It will examine the currently available technologies and those in the pipeline and discuss the opportunities and challenges to answer to the unique healthcare needs of migrant populations, the barriers they face in accessing traditional services, and the innovative approaches being used to integrate POC

V. Padovese (✉)
Bridges2Health&Rights NGO, Msida, Malta

Genitourinary Clinic, Department of Dermatology and Venereology, Mater Dei Hospital, Msida, Malta
e-mail: valeska.padovese@gov.mt

K. Blondeel
Faculty of Medicine and Health Sciences, Ghent University, Ghent, Belgium
e-mail: karel.blondeel@ugent.be

V. Padovese, I. Rossoni (eds.), *Intersections of Sexual Health, Migration and Sexualised Violence*, Sustainable Development Goals Series, https://doi.org/10.1007/978-3-032-20707-4_10

testing into community-based sexual health programs. We will also discuss some cautionary measures so that POCT is implemented in a way that maximizes the potential of these technologies to improve health outcomes, reduce the spread of STIs, and empower individuals in vulnerable situations to take control of their sexual health.

Keywords

POCT · Sexual health · STIs · HIV · Migrants · Refugees

10.1 Background

10.1.1 Global Burden of STIs

Sexually transmitted infections (STIs), including HIV, remain a major global public health challenge (Implementing the global health sector strategies on HIV, viral hepatitis and sexually transmitted infections, 2022–2030: report on progress and gaps 2024). Each day, more than one million cases of four curable STIs—syphilis (*Treponema pallidum*), gonorrhoea (*Neisseria gonorrhoeae*), chlamydia (*Chlamydia trachomatis*), and trichomoniasis (*Trichomonas vaginalis*)—are reported worldwide (Sexually transmitted infections (STIs) 2024).

In 2022, WHO Member States set an ambitious goal to reduce adult syphilis infections by tenfold by 2030, targeting a drop from 7.1 million cases in 2020 to 0.71 million (Global health sector strategies on HIV, viral hepatitis and sexually transmitted infections for the period 2022–2030 2024). However, new syphilis cases among adults aged 15–49 rose by over one million in 2022, reaching a total of eight million, with the highest increases observed in the Americas and African region (Global and regional STI estimates 2024).

Notably, new data indicate an alarming rise in multi-resistant gonorrhoea. Among the 87 countries with enhanced gonorrhoea antimicrobial resistance surveillance in 2023, 9 reported increased resistance (>= 5%) to ceftriaxone, currently the last-line treatment for gonorrhoea (Implementing the global health sector strategies on HIV, viral hepatitis and sexually transmitted infections, 2022–2030: report on progress and gaps 2024).

STIs cause a high burden of morbidity and mortality, particularly in low- and middle-income countries (LMICs), impacting the quality of life of adults and, as a result of vertical transmission, of infants and children (Vargas et al. 2022). Additionally, they also facilitate the sexual transmission of HIV by increasing both the susceptibility to HIV infection and infectiousness of those persons who are already co-infected.

Between 2020 and 2022, new HIV infections declined only modestly, from 1.5 million to 1.3 million (Implementing the global health sector strategies on HIV, viral hepatitis and sexually transmitted infections, 2022–2030: report on progress and gaps 2024). Five key population groups—men who have sex with men, people who inject drugs, sex workers, transgender individuals, and individuals in prisons and other closed settings—continue to face significantly higher HIV incidence rates than the general population (Korenromp et al. 2024). These groups and their partners account for an estimated 55% of new HIV infections. HIV-related mortality remains high, with 630,000 deaths recorded in 2022; notably, 13% of these deaths were among children under 15 (Implementing the global health sector strategies on HIV, viral hepatitis and sexually transmitted infections, 2022–2030: report on progress and gaps 2024).

10.1.2 Burden of STIs in Migrant Populations

Migrant populations, following the definition of the International Organization for Migration (IOM), include all persons who move away from their place of usual residence, whether within a country or across an international border, temporarily or permanently, for a variety of reasons. This includes a number of well-defined legal categories of people, but also some groups of people whose status or means of movement are not specifically defined under international law.

Some migrant populations seem to be more vulnerable to STIs, including HIV, compared to non-migrants. According to a European Centre for Disease Prevention and Control (ECDC) report from 2023, migrants (defined as 'people born abroad') are a key population affected by HIV across Europe and Central Asia, accounting for 42% of new HIV diagnoses in the European Economic Area (EEA) in 2021 and 48% of those diagnosed in 2022 (HIV and migrants – Monitoring the implementation of the Dublin Declaration on partnership to fight HIV/AIDS in Europe and Central Asia: 2022 progress report 2023). A systematic review including more than seven million migrants, including foreign born migrants, refugees, undocumented migrants, and asylum seekers, showed that globally, the HIV prevalence ratio was higher among migrants than in native-born populations (Santoso et al. 2022). Some migrants may come from countries with higher population-based national prevalence of HIV, but increased rates of HIV transmission in refugee and migrant populations have also been observed due to forced displacement, particularly along border areas and transportation routes (Cortes et al. 2024). Moreover, migrants, after having migrated, seem to be more likely than non-migrants to acquire HIV in their new countries of residence, often due to increased vulnerability in host countries, along with barriers to accessing healthcare services (Migration, Human Mobility and HIV 2024; Mann et al. 2024). Data from the HIV prevention response seems to highlight the disparity in service access; indicative of a gap in prevention services, only a handful of European countries were able to report substantial pre-exposure prophylaxis (PrEP) uptake among migrants (Monitoring HIV pre-exposure prophylaxis programmes in the EU/EEA 2022). Additionally, only a minority of countries have comprehensive data tracking the HIV care continuum—diagnosis, treatment, and viral suppression—among foreign-born individuals.

Migrant populations are not being mentioned in WHO's most recent progress and gap report following the global health sector strategies on HIV, viral hepatitis, and STIs (Implementing the global health sector strategies on HIV, viral hepatitis and sexually transmitted infections, 2022–2030: report on progress and gaps 2024). There is very scarce and dispersed data of the epidemiology of STIs, as global HIV/STI surveillance among these populations faces ethical and logistical challenges, but there has been a noticeable increase in diagnoses of some STIs (Panchenko et al. 2024). In some countries, this increase is especially apparent on the intersection of migrant status and other vulnerabilities; in Malta for example among foreign-born gay and bisexual men, cases have risen by 36% over the past decade. This underscores the importance of targeting key populations within migrant populations with effective sexual health interventions (Padovese et al. 2021).

10.1.3 Barriers to Accessing Sexual Health Services in Migrant Populations

Although international human rights agreements guarantee the universal right to healthcare, including sexual healthcare, for migrant and refugee populations, the Sustainable Development Goals do not contain any specific indicator on health and migration (New York Declaration for Refugees and Migrants 2024; Global Compact on Refugees 2017; Mosler Vidal et al. 2022). There is a multitude of barriers for migrants to accessing sexual health services on individual, interpersonal, and societal levels; moreover, systemic challenges prevent migrant populations from attaining sexual well-being (Panchenko et al. 2024). Personal-level barriers include, for instance, psychological stress and trauma stemming from migration experience knowledge, low health (STI prevention) literacy, economic or geographical barriers, fear of legal consequences or a lack of trust in healthcare services, and earlier negative experiences (Panchenko et al. 2024). On the interpersonal level, cultural and language barriers may result in poor communication with healthcare providers and poor care experiences. This may be exacerbated by societal level impact of stigma and discrimination, specifically for STIs, as migrant populations may be accused of having 'imported' these infections to the non-migrant population (Irons 2022). This stigma may intersect with other forms of stigma and discrimination based on gender identity, sexual orientation, sex work, or socioeconomic status, further limiting access to (sexual) healthcare services. Organizational and structural barriers include health system factors such as the lack of entitlement to health services, often depending on migration status, restricted access to health insurance, and the unaffordable cost of medicine particularly in non-universal health systems (Gil-González et al. 2015; Mitjà et al. 2023). Further, migrant health is structurally underfunded and migrants are often systemically pushed into poor living and working conditions (Lebano et al. 2020).

Often called "hard to reach," this may seem to put the responsibility for the lack of access with the service receiver, not recognizing that people are not getting the services and support they need. The exclusion of migrant populations from health services often stems from a lack of political engagement and appropriate approaches, increasing their risk to poor health outcomes. This highlights the importance of targeted policy-making and planning to address structural challenges, provide comprehensive STI care, and the need of improving STI-knowledge, testing, and early service utilization among migrants (Mitjà et al. 2023).

10.2 Point-of-Care Testing (POCT) for STIs Including HIV

Early diagnosis of STIs, including HIV, is critical not only for individual health but also for preventing the transmission of infections within and between communities. With some exceptions, diagnostic approaches typically require multiple visits to healthcare facilities, laboratory testing by skilled technicians, and prolonged waiting periods for results, and are ill suited to many low-resource settings and the needs of migrant populations.

Syndromic management—providing treatment based on a patient's symptoms and clinical signs, such as urethral or vaginal discharge and genital ulcer disease—has long been recommended as a way to address challenges related to loss to follow-up and the cost of diagnostic testing. However, many STIs do not have unique presentations or may be asymptomatic, leading to both overtreatment which may increase antimicrobial resistance and undertreatment (Vargas et al. 2022). Therefore, the most recent WHO global health sector strategy for STIs promotes a transition from syndromic management to aetiologic testing, both for case management and screening (World Health Organization 2022). Testing at the point-of-care (POC) allows to move aetiology-based diagnosis from centralized laboratories to primary health centres, close to where patients seek healthcare. STI point-of-care testing, in addition to enabling diagnosis and appropriate treatment or referral in a single visit, also often enables self-collection of samples (see Box 10.1) and paves the way for innovative STI-service delivery methods, such as non-clinical site delivery, community- and home-based testing (including screening), as well as self-testing (see Box 10.2). POC tests have also been shown to be cost-effective compared with alternatives such as syndromic management and laboratory diagnosis (World Health Organization 2023).

In 2006, WHO introduced the ASSURED criteria for POC tests: affordable, sensitive, specific, user-friendly, rapid and robust, equipment-free, and deliverable to end users. Following a recent landscape analysis, there is still a lack of STI POC tests that comply with all these criteria (The diagnostics landscape for sexually transmitted infections 2024). In response, WHO has published target product profiles (TPPs), indicating minimal and preferred characteristics for a multitude of test parameters, to assure tests under development better fit the global health needs (Point-of-care tests for sexually transmitted infections: target product profiles 2024). Partly inspired by the COVID-pandemic, there have been recent technological advances in point-of-care testing that do hold promise for truly affordable STI POC tests. These can assist, as they have already proven, in providing sexual health services that are accessible and inclusive for currently underserved populations such as migrants. The WHO global research priorities exercise for STIs showed that the top four STI research areas were related to development and implementation of low-cost, rapid POC tests, especially in LMICs (Gottlieb et al. 2024).

While POC testing has emerged as a transformative tool in sexual healthcare, offering new opportunities to reach underserved populations, it has also spurred debate among specialists, clinicians, primary health workers, laboratory technicians, public health experts, and policy-makers regarding the appropriate use and quality control, particularly in resource-constrained settings.

Box 10.1 Self-sampling

Self-sampling enables individuals to collect their own biological samples, such as urine, oral, pharyngeal, vaginal, or anal swabs, both at the POC or at home, which may be instantaneously analysed with a POC test or sent to a laboratory for analysis. This method is frequently used to detect infections like chlamydia, gonorrhoea, and the human papillomavirus (HPV). By allowing samples to be sent by mail, self-sampling removes barriers related to stigma, inconvenience, or distance from clinics, offering a more private way to get tested. This discretion encourages people who might otherwise avoid clinic visits. In the event of a positive result, follow-up can be arranged through telemedicine, and treatment may be prescribed and sent by email or phone apps without the need for in-person clinic visits. Studies show that self-sampling increases testing rates, particularly among underserved groups and those who may avoid traditional settings due to stigma or privacy concerns such as young people, sex workers, and men who have sex with men. It can also be integrated into outreach services to extend testing to remote or hard-to-reach areas. Even in conventional screening pathways, self-sampling may increase testing rates. Studies have further shown that self-collected samples have the same quality as provider collected samples (Taylor et al. 2013).

Box 10.2 Self-testing

Self-testing is not to be confused with self-collection of samples as it goes a step further by allowing individuals to obtain instantaneous results without involvement of a health care provider or a laboratory. Self-testing kits, particularly for HIV, have become increasingly popular, delivering rapid results within 20–40 minutes. A key advantage of self-testing is the immediate feedback it provides, which can prompt timely actions like seeking care, adjusting behaviours to reduce transmission risks, and encouraging screening among individuals who may avoid traditional testing settings due to stigma or privacy concerns.

However, implementing self-testing presents some challenges. For example, individuals must understand how to interpret their results accurately and know what steps to take next, particularly if the result is reactive (positive). Ensuring that those who receive positive results connect with healthcare providers for confirmatory testing, counselling, and treatment is essential. Additionally, receiving a positive result alone at home can be distressing, so it's crucial to provide clear guidance on follow-up support.

Self-testing, particularly for HIV, has shown promising results in increasing diagnosis rates in at-risk populations. For example, HIV self-testing has been particularly impactful in sub-Saharan Africa, where access to healthcare can be limited, and stigma associated with clinic-based

(continued)

testing may deter individuals (Hacking et al. 2022).

Research is ongoing for developing reliable self-tests for other STIs and to integrate self-sampling and self-testing with digital tools, such as apps that offer counselling or follow-up support, improving linkage to care and adherence to treatment. If used appropriately and rolled-out after validation and piloting in the context where it will be used, self-testing is a promising, patient-centred approach that may improve accessibility, reduce stigma, and facilitate early diagnosis. When combined with digital health innovations and strong healthcare support networks, it can make significant contributions to sexual health and STI-related outcomes (Liu et al. 2019; Venter et al. 2018).

10.2.1 Currently Available STI POC Tests

We follow the description of a POC test published previously as an affordable test that can be performed by a non-laboratory trained health worker and/or lay health worker, outside of a laboratory setting at the site at which clinical care is being provided, and where test results are generally made available on the same day as sample collection and testing, to enable clinical decisions to be made in a timely manner (World Health Organization 2024). This description can accommodate—tests utilizing various technologies and in a variety of formats—for example, lateral flow tests, similar to pregnancy tests in format or molecular tests. Moreover, the POC test concept is not only determined by technology but also by context and the end-users (Toskin et al. 2017a).

The first lateral flow HIV tests have been available since the early 1990s, and currently such POC tests for syphilis, both treponemal and/or non-treponemal, and dual HIV/syphilis tests exhibit adequate performance and acceptability, as does one such test for trichomonas vaginalis (Adamson et al. 2020). However, for chlamydia and gonorrhoeae, this type of test suffers from low diagnostic sensitivity, which makes it unfit for screening purposes (Grillo-Ardila et al. 2020). Moreover, most lateral flow tests are read with the naked eye, which makes its interpretation subjective and dependent on factors such as lighting conditions, user training, and patient flow.

Molecular amplification testing methods (nucleic acid amplification tests or NAATs), which detect specific sequences of DNA or RNA, have substantially changed the microbiological diagnosis of pathogens and have in many cases become the gold standard or test of choice for among others chlamydia and gonorrhoea. Some of the commercially available NAATs may be used at the point of care to overcome the performance limitations of lateral flow tests, while maintaining rapidity and offering real-time connectivity. However, they are not yet equipment-free and are generally too expensive for routine implementation in most LMICs (World Health Organization 2023).

The World Health Organisation (WHO) has published several diagnostic landscapes with commercially available STI POC tests, including references to publications on their performance, the last one dating from 2023 (The diagnostics landscape for sexually transmitted infections 2025). Additionally, WHO regularly updates its list of pre-qualified in vitro diagnostics, meaning that they meet WHO standards, to assist procurers with both quality assurance and product selection (Prequalified In Vitro Diagnostics | WHO 2025). It should be noted that WHO prequalification is manufacturer initiated.

Over the years many new tests have been on the horizon but have never made to the market or have never been evaluated thoroughly. It has now been over 10 years since the first target product profiles (TPPs) for STI POC tests were published by the WHO, guiding manufacturers on the characteristics required to meet public health needs. However, no chlamydia or gonorrhoea test currently meets the minimal criteria, indicating that the prioritization of STI POC diagnostics—excluding HIV and, to some extent, syphilis—remains relatively low despite the urgent need for accurate screening and treatment. (Toskin et al.

2017a; Point-of-care tests for sexually transmitted infections: target product profiles 2024).

10.2.2 Technological Advances in STI POC Testing

Apart from the availability of well-validated POC tests, the lack of affordable tests is a critical barrier to widespread implementation of STI-screening. Ideally the technology of an STI POC test should be self-contained, fully integrated sample-to-report, allow for raw, untreated specimens, perform all molecular steps, and provide interpreted test results in less than 30 minutes.

There is some promise to achieve this as the pipeline of STI diagnostics has undergone a rapid transformation, driven by general advancements in diagnostic technologies and COVID-19-related innovations, showing among other things that solutions can be achieved quickly when are thought to be required and when funding is available (Manabe 2023). The COVID-19 pandemic has demonstrated that developing cost-effective and flexible yet reliable diagnostic tests is possible (Poljak et al. 2021).

One promising approach is the use of isothermal amplification technologies such as loop-mediated isothermal amplification (LAMP), which can provide results under an hour. There have been LAMP-based products developed, but these still needs an instrument and includes several manual operator steps; moreover, they have not been commercialized as of yet (Dean et al. 2021; Rodriguez-Mateos et al. 2023; Esitgen Germaner et al. 2023; Liu et al. 2017). To decrease cost, technologies for reading of the test results with the naked eye, with or without electrochemical signal enhancement, have been proposed, as have modified LAMP technologies, promising to be cheap, rapid, and sensitive (Tanner et al. 2015; Tayyab et al. 2023). Recombinase polymerase amplification (RPA), another isothermal amplification technology, may provide quick test results and allow for multiplexing (Zhang et al. 2025; Fan et al. 2023). RPA reactions can be performed within a temperature range of 25–42 °C and RPA reagents can be lyophilized, enabling long-term storage and transportation and paper-based techniques (Fang et al. 2025). Additionally, emerging highly specific CRISPR-Cas-based test technologies are gaining attention for their potential to be used on biochips integrated with everyday technology, such as mobile phones, which can provide power, processing, and result display functions (Zhou et al. 2025; Yang et al. 2024). With the advent of biosensors—small devices that use biological reactions to detect target analytes—lateral flow techniques are re-emerging as promising diagnostic tools (Chen et al. 2022).

Recent advances in microfluidics-based POC test technology such as paper, array, and beads have shown promising results for diagnosing various infectious diseases, further minimizing the need for instruments, which use capillary action to transport fluids without pumps, valves, or other fluid handling equipment (Rodriguez et al. 2016; Kumar et al. 2022). These paper-based systems are eco-friendly, easy to use, and practically equipment-free, making them ideal for remote or underserved areas.

Future directions include exploring enzyme-DNA nanostructures, digital hybridization, and single-cell droplet PCR methods that may eventually bypass the need for DNA amplification altogether, paving the way for a new era of POC diagnostics (Zhang et al. 2020). These new technologies should be integrated with AI-assisted STI screening tools for symptomatic patients (Soe et al. 2025).

These innovations could revolutionize STI screening by enabling faster, more affordable, and thus more accessible STI tests. As with currently available STI tests, these innovative tests should be thoroughly clinically validated and piloted, and be readily available on the market, before they can be rolled out. There has been exponential growth in POC–related publications for infectious diseases in general. Improved public awareness, stronger healthcare team coordination, and early planning for POC testing at entry points—including among migrant populations—will be crucial to maximizing societal benefit (Sweileh 2024).

10.3 Implementation of STI POCTs Among Migrant Populations

10.3.1 Implementation Experiences and Case Study

As mentioned above, migrant populations may face higher risks of STI infection due to various factors related to their situation both in the country or region of origin, and their current location, including in humanitarian settings, the transient nature of their stay, and migratory experience (Vasylyeva et al. 2022; Jordan et al. 2021). Suboptimal health-seeking behaviour combined with lack of access to sexual health services averts them from receiving timely diagnosis and treatment, resulting in many infections remaining undetected and untreated. POC may thus assist in providing rapid, accurate results, allowing for immediate diagnosis and/or linkage to care in a variety of settings related to migration.

STI POC tests have been deployed successfully in different settings, although mostly for HIV and syphilis, depending on their relatively low cost and availability. A recent evidence synthesis on interventions to ensure access to and continuity of HIV care for international migrants identified utilization of mobile health, mobile units, and community-led initiatives to bring HIV care to migrants (Kamenshchikova et al. 2024).

In Greece, one of the current technologies that can be used at the POC for NG and CT was used among migrants, and although it came out more expensive in direct costs compared to syndromic management, it is beneficial to decrease antimicrobial resistance (and costs) in the long term, as far less people were unnecessarily treated (Tsorou et al. 2024). Because of the transient nature of migrant populations, often located in underserved areas, it is important to use the least invasive sampling methods; for Bangladesh, for example, the use of POC oral fluid tests for HIV has shown to successfully enable the assessment of HIV prevalence in rural-based returnee migrants (Alam et al. 2016).

Box 10.3 describes a forthcoming project across three Southern European countries that will build on STI POC technologies for better sexual health outcomes in migrant communities.

Box 10.3 Case Example: REACH-OUT Project Malta, Italy, and Greece

Italy, Malta, and Greece are the gateways to Europe's Southern border. These countries have witnessed a steady rise in migration flows in recent years, with migrants, asylum-seekers, and refugees reaching their borders through the Central, Eastern Mediterranean, and Balkan routes. Project "REACH-OUT" originated from field experiences of the involved partners, who are providing health services to individuals pushed to the margin of society: undocumented migrants, refugees and asylum seekers, impoverished locals, and many other "disadvantaged" individuals. These groups lack access to structural prevention initiatives that are culturally sensitive; have limited awareness about STIs, HIV, and hepatitis; and lack access to information concerning HIV preventative interventions.

The project intends to decrease incidence of HIV/AIDS, tuberculosis and STIs, by offering direct services to end users; disseminating easily understandable and accessible information on prevention, care, treatment; and lastly by improving and supporting both institutional capacity and response.

The overall objective of the project is to improve health outcomes for migrants and disadvantaged local population groups through prevention, early detection, and access to care for tuberculosis, HIV, STIs, hepatitis B and C in Italy, Malta, and Greece, and to reinforce and promote stakeholders' cooperation.

(continued)

Project Goals

The REACH-OUT project implements a range of initiatives aimed at enhancing outreach efforts for migrant and refugee populations, with particular focus on the vulnerability of the situation in the country of origin. The goal is to promote early testing via the use of POC testing, improve health service access, and ensure that outreach and awareness-raising efforts are consistent, standardized across Europe, and grounded in evidence. This approach actively involves key social actors: end users (migrants, refugees, and other disadvantaged individuals, including locals), institutions (health and local authorities), and NGOs working in the field. In addition, the project includes specific actions to raise awareness and promote HIV/AIDS and tuberculosis prevention to broad audiences, including the general public, migrant communities, healthcare professionals, institutions, and organizations, to maximize impact. A holistic approach is adopted, integrating internet technology and social media to deliver a targeted communication campaign using platforms popular among migrant populations.

REACH-OUT's specific objectives include:

- *Improving Access to Testing and Care*: Expanding early testing opportunities and healthcare access for migrants, refugees, and disadvantaged local groups, including third-country nationals, men who have sex with men, transgender individuals, and sex workers, to ensure no community is left behind.
- *Raising Awareness of Preventative Health Practices*: Education preventive health and behaviours to reduce transmission of infections and promote overall health and well-being.
- *Capacity-Building and Best Practices Exchange*: Facilitating the development of skills, knowledge, and resources across countries, enabling national and transnational partners to share and implement best practices effectively.
- *Fostering Multi-level, Multi-stakeholder Cooperation*: Creating a collaborative network involving various stakeholders at different levels to address sexual health and tuberculosis issues comprehensively within the most vulnerable populations.
- *Conducting Evidence-Based Research*: Using research to drive evidence-based interventions and to monitor, evaluate, and adapt the project's methods for maximal effectiveness.

By addressing the complex healthcare challenges faced by migrant and refugee populations, REACH-OUT is committed to advancing health equity, reducing healthcare disparities, and fostering resilient health systems across Europe.

Results and Impact

The REACH-OUT project aims to bring about several key changes:

- *Behavioural Change in Health Practices:* Encourage healthier behaviours among target groups, particularly concerning HIV/STI prevention and care, through education and awareness.
- *Improved Access to Public Health Services:* Increase attendance and improve access to public health services, ensuring that even the most marginalized individuals can receive necessary care.
- *Enhanced Capacity for Health Authorities:* Support health authorities in effectively reaching all residents within their jurisdictions, including undocumented individuals and those living in informal settlements.

(continued)

- *Expanded Knowledge Among Trainees:* Strengthen the knowledge and skills of trained professionals, equipping them with practical tools for effective outreach.
- *Improved Psychological Support for Service Providers:* Enhance the capacity of psychological support providers to manage emotionally demanding situations, reducing burnout and ensuring sustainable, compassionate care.

Role of STI POC testing

STI point-of-care (POC) testing plays a central role in the Reach Out project by enabling early detection, rapid treatment, and effective prevention of sexually transmitted infections within the community. Because POC tests deliver results within minutes, they help reduce barriers to care—especially for individuals who may not return for follow-up visits or who face stigma, transportation issues, or limited access to healthcare. Moreover, individuals who test positive can be counselled immediately and referred/linked to care to start treatment promptly. By treating infections quickly, POCT directly contributes to lowering transmission rates, strengthen community trust, and engagement.

10.3.2 Benefits and Promises of STI POC Testing Among Migrants

10.3.2.1 Rapid Results and Immediate Treatment

The immediate advantage of deploying POC tests in clinical setting is the enabling of a "one-stop-shop" facilitating results and treatment and or referral in a single visit. This is particularly crucial for migrant populations in vulnerable situations, where delays in obtaining results may lead to loss to follow-up leading to increased health complications and potential further transmission of STIs in the community. Immediate access to treatment or referral not only improves individual health outcomes but also helps to mitigate the broader public health impact of STIs.

10.3.2.2 Reduction of Stigma and Culturally Sensitive Care

Traditional STI testing often requires patients to visit centralized healthcare facilities, which may be culturally unwelcoming for hard-to-reach populations. POC testing can be conducted in various settings—such as community health centres, outreach programs, mobile clinics, and even pharmacies—making it easier for individuals to get tested without facing barriers related to the stigma they may face associated with seeking sexual health services. By offering testing in less formal and more private settings, POC testing can foster a more comfortable environment, encouraging individuals from migrant communities or in humanitarian settings to seek necessary care without fear of judgment.

10.3.2.3 Patient Empowerment and Engagement

POC testing often involves self-sampling options, which empower individuals to take control of their sexual health. This empowerment is particularly important for hard-to-reach populations, as it encourages proactive engagement with their health. For HIV, syphilis, and hepatitis C, there are self-testing options, enabling an individual to collect their specimen using a simple rapid diagnostic test, perform the test, interpret their result, and share their result with a healthcare provider when and where they want. Empowerment through self-testing may also enhance health literacy and reduce feelings of helplessness.

10.3.2.4 Cost-Effectiveness

POC testing may be more cost-effective compared to traditional laboratory testing methods, as they reduce the need for extensive laboratory infrastructure and staffing. This is particularly beneficial in resource-limited settings where funds are scarce. Lower costs can facilitate broader implementation of testing programs, ensuring that services are more accessible to hard-to-reach areas and communities.

10.3.2.5 Integration with Other Services

POC testing may easily be integrated with other health services, such as harm reduction programs, family planning for migrant women, substance use, or general health screenings. This integrated approach can streamline healthcare delivery, making it easier for individuals to access a comprehensive range of services in one visit.

10.3.2.6 Addressing Public Health Goals

The use of POC testing aligns with broader public health goals, including reducing STI transmission rates and achieving the World Health Organization's (WHO) targets for STI management. By increasing access to testing in key populations, health authorities can enhance surveillance efforts, allowing for more effective response strategies and resource allocation. Moreover, new pathways incorporating POC molecular testing in symptomatic patients may improve the precision of antibiotic prescribing and reduce unnecessary use (Wong et al. 2024).

10.3.2.7 Decentralizing of Testing

POCT technologies can be used in non-clinical settings such as community outreach programs, mobile clinics, pharmacies, effectively bypassing the barriers associated with traditional healthcare facilities. The portability, ease of use, and low cost of these technologies make them particularly well suited to ensure that even the most isolated or stigmatized individuals can receive the care they need (Banfi et al. 2024).

10.3.3 Challenges and Attention Points

10.3.3.1 Technical Limitations and Validation

While technical advances will potentially change the game for STI POC testing, all tests should be independently validated in the laboratory not only under ideal circumstances but also under real life conditions, integrated in a clinical or non-clinical setting. Feasibility and acceptability to both providers and health users should be evaluated. Several studies have shown that performance in the field is a lot lower than in controlled environments and can differ depending on the context in which they are used (Cordioli et al. 2024; Sherriff et al. 2024; Shephard et al. 2024a; Kularatne et al. 2024). This is especially relevant for using POC tests in migrant populations.

10.3.3.2 Infrastructure Challenges

Decentralized testing may increase accessibility of the services and follow-up but places pressure on health systems, particularly in terms, infrastructure, and human resources (Toskin et al. 2017b). In some settings where there is a concentration of migrant populations, such as humanitarian settings or underserved marginal areas, storage, electricity, and cold-chain (if needed) may be absent and supply may be non-continuous. Some of these obstacles may be overcome by choosing the right kind of test, but technology will not be the only answer.

10.3.3.3 Regulatory and Legal Issues

Although some ISO standards have been established, standards and regulations can vary not only between regions and countries but also across different healthcare settings. Variability may concern aspects such as self-sampling and self-testing, which (non-)medical professionals are permitted to collect or analyze samples, who is authorized to communicate results to patients, and who can decide on, prescribe, administer treatment, or provide referrals. A POC test and its use should be adapted to these standards and regulations, or, if evidence-based, organizations may advocate to have amended regulations for extraordinary circumstances.

10.3.3.4 Quality Control

Though the operator steps of POC may seem straightforward, they remain, as every test, vulnerable to errors. These errors may originate from, among other things, manufacturing or storage issues, specimen collection or transport (preanalytical), test operators, specimen reagent interaction (intra-analytical), reporting, interpreting, and recording results (post-analytical) (Chitneni et al. 2023). While POC test may overcome some of these issues (if a patient wait for the results, they don't have to be called back), they may also be more challenging (if a patient who is, for example, a transient migrant is not able to wait for the results, treatment is not available, or referral is needed, how will they be followed up?).

For a start, concepts of good clinical laboratory practice should be known to all providers involved in POC testing. Internal quality control (IQC) and external quality assurance (EQA) should also be inherent parts of POC testing. Although assays may have some (but not all) internal quality controls, some do not and POC test settings should be assisted by laboratories to set up IQC procedures. The most common EQA method, to control the quality of testing at a certain site, is external proficiency testing, whereby a reference laboratory distributes and gives performance feedback on blinded proficiency testing panels analysed by POC sites (Cao et al. 2024; Shephard et al. 2024b). Given the mobility of certain migrant populations, many envisioned POC testing sites may lack these quality procedures or the know-how to set them up. This may increase time and cost to set up quality STI POC test services.

10.3.3.5 Training and Education

As stated above, the quality of testing is also dependent on the providers. Shortages and high turnover of health care providers, combined with the lack of capacity of a laboratory to train and monitor laboratory and non-laboratory health workers included in POC testing at the sites, may complicate the roll out of POC testing. In underserved communities such as migrants, it is all the more important that experiences with healthcare are positive. Health care providers and community health workers alike should be trained on migrant inclusive care (including context specific religious and cultural considerations) and be experts in and proponents of POC testing, for STI POC services to succeed.

10.3.3.6 Cost

POC testing is not necessarily cheaper than laboratory testing. If quality laboratory services are accessible and efficient, it may be more costly to set up and sustain POC testing, meaning that other services in the health system may be endangered, or other groups may be denied health services. The cost, supply, and maintenance of POC technology and reagents, along with the ongoing training of personnel in low- and middle-income countries (LMICs) or remote areas—often with higher proportions of migrant populations—are likely higher than in urban, high-income settings.

10.3.3.7 Ethical Considerations

Medical pathways should be anticipated before introducing STI POC testing. Firstly, if sustained availability of treatments cannot be guaranteed, testing may be less ethical than not testing. Secondly, testing and counselling should always happen with full consent and in confidentiality. Some of the barriers mentioned above can make it challenging to assure such circumstances. Thirdly, although POC tests should enable same visit results, time to treatment may take longer than, for example, syndromic management, or take away time for other medical appointments or treatments, potentially burdening the patient (Chitneni et al. 2023). Fourthly, there should be attention for not overburdening the healthcare provider, both in regular and humanitarian settings. Opportunistically adding an STI POC test to a regular visit may unnecessarily increase their time per patient and their responsibility concerning medical decisions.

Lastly, if STI POC services are available to the general population, they should be made available to migrant populations. Likewise, it could also be ethically challenging if STI POC initiatives would be available to migrant populations but not to other people inhabiting the same area.

10.3.4 No Size Fits All

Within a country or region, or even within an area serviced by a health centre, POC and non-POC testing may go hand in hand for STIs, depending on the public, location, and the context. Within the STI POC concept, there are also different delivery methods that may be used to reach underserved migrant communities. These strategies may include a combination of community-based approaches, such as partnering with community organizations (Kamenshchikova et al. 2024) and peer navigators, using culturally sensitive materials and translation services, mobile outreach (Townsend et al. 2024) and pop-up testing sites, integrating sexual health services with harm reduction programs or shelters, and leveraging non-traditional settings—such as pharmacies (Figueira et al. 2022), hair salons, barber shops, social clubs, sporting events, or "hotspots" for sexual activity.

Interventions may need to be tailored to specific subgroups of migrant populations, for example by employing gender-sensitive approaches—particularly to address the needs of women and sexual and gender minority migrants—offering services outside normal working hours, or combining telehealth with self-testing. To sustain an efficient combination of these delivery methods, there should be a both sturdy and flexible health system in place.

10.4 Conclusion

In summary, POC testing offers significant advantages in addressing the unique healthcare needs of migrant populations. By overcoming barriers to access, reducing stigma, and providing rapid results, these testing methods represent a critical component of effective sexual health interventions if their introduction has been well prepared. Their integration into healthcare strategies can help ensure that even the most marginalized individuals receive the care they need, ultimately contributing to improved public health outcomes.

While healthcare systems continue to grapple with the dual challenges of STI prevention and equitable access, near-future STI POC technologies hold a promise to produce reliable tests at a fraction of the current cost. Policy makers, developers, and manufacturers, both public and private, should be called upon to hold the promise for bridging the gap between underserved migrant populations and essential sexual healthcare services.

References

Adamson PC, Loeffelholz MJ, Klausner JD (2020) Point-of-care testing for sexually transmitted infections a review of recent developments. Arch Pathol Lab Med 144:1344–1351

Alam MS, Khan SI, Reza M, Shahriar A, Sarker MS, Rahman A et al (2016) Point of care HIV testing with oral fluid among returnee migrants in a rural area of Bangladesh. Curr Opin HIV AIDS 11(Suppl 1):S52–S58

Banfi G, Božič B, Cihan M, Pašalić D, Pennestrì F, Plebani M (2024) Point-of-care testing, near-patient testing and patient self-testing: warning points. Clin Chem Lab Med CCLM 62:2388–2392

Cao W, Fakile YF, Shukla MR, Pettus K, Lupoli K, Hong J et al (2024) External quality assessment to support the WHO ProSPeRo study for the evaluation of two dual HIV/syphilis point-of-care tests in seven countries. BMC Infect Dis 24:194

Chen X, Yuan W, Zhou Q, Tan Y, Wang R, Dong S (2022) Sensitive and visual identification of Chlamydia trachomatis using multiple cross displacement amplification integrated with a gold nanoparticle-based lateral flow biosensor for point-of-care use. Front Cell Infect Microbiol 12. https://doi.org/10.3389/fcimb.2022.949514

Chitneni P, Owembabazi M, Muyindike W, Asiimwe S, Masete G, Mbalibulha Y et al (2023) Sexually transmitted infection point-of-care testing in resource-limited settings: a narrative review guided by an implementation framework. Sex Transm Dis 50:e11–e16

Cordioli M, Gios L, Erbogasto A, Mirandola M, Sandri A, Padovese V et al (2024) Clinic-based evaluation of the dual Xpert CT/NG assay on the GeneXpert system for screening for extragenital chlamydial and gonococcal infections amongst men who have sex with men. BMC Infect Dis 24:224

Cortes CP, Sued O, Wong WCW, Borquez A, Ssonko C, Parczewski M et al (2024) Humanising and optimising HIV health care for refugees and asylum seekers. Lancet HIV 11:e861–e872

Dean D, Swaminathan S, Kama M, Goemans S, Faktaufon D, Alnabelseya N et al (2021) Development and evaluation of a point-of-care test in a low-resource setting with high rates of Chlamydia trachomatis urogenital infections in Fiji. J Clin Microbiol 59:e00182–21

Esitgen Germaner ET, Wassill L, Dichtl K, Roider J, Seybold U (2023) Rapid point of care testing for four bacterial sexually transmitted infections using the portable isothermal loop-mediated nucleic acid amplification eazyplex platform. Infection 51:1141–1145

Fan M, Yang J, Wang X, Xu Y, Li B, Yang H et al (2023) Highly specific detection of *Neisseria gonorrhoeae* based on recombinase polymerase amplification-initiated strand displacement amplification. Anal Chim Acta 1283:341956

Fang F, Guo H, Guo Z, Lin L, Lai L, Shi Y et al (2025) A simple and colorimetric method utilizing cell-free toehold switch sensors for the detection of *Chlamydia trachomatis*, *Ureaplasma urealyticum* and *Neisseria gonorrhoeae*. Anal Chim Acta 1339:343622

Figueira I, Teixeira I, Rodrigues AT, Gama A, Dias S (2022) Point-of-care HIV and hepatitis screening in community pharmacies: a quantitative and qualitative study. Int J Clin Pharm 44:1158–1168

Gil-González D, Carrasco-Portiño M, Vives-Cases C, Agudelo-Suárez AA, Castejón Bolea R, Ronda-Pérez E (2015) Is health a right for all? An umbrella review of the barriers to health care access faced by migrants. Ethn Health 20:523–541

Global and regional STI estimates [web site] (https://www.who.int/data/gho/data/themes/topics/global-and-regional-sti-estimates, Accessed 10 Dec 2024)

Global Compact on Refugees [web site] (2017) (https://refugeesmigrants.un.org/refugees-compact, Accessed 18 Dec 2024)

Global health sector strategies on HIV, viral hepatitis and sexually transmitted infections for the period 2022–2030 [web site] (https://www.who.int/publications/i/item/9789240053779, Accessed 10 Dec 2024)

Gottlieb SL, Spielman E, Abu-Raddad L, Aderoba AK, Bachmann LH, Blondeel K et al (2024) WHO global research priorities for sexually transmitted infections. Lancet Glob Health 12:e1544–e1551

Grillo-Ardila CF, Torres M, Gaitán HG (2020) Rapid point of care test for detecting urogenital chlamydia trachomatis infection in nonpregnant women and men at reproductive age. Cochrane Database Syst Rev 2020:CD011708

Hacking D, Cassidy T, Ellman T, Steele SJ, Moore HA, Bermudez-Aza E et al (2022) HIV self-testing among previously diagnosed HIV-positive people in Khayelitsha, South Africa: no evidence of harm but may facilitate re-engagement in ART care. AIDS Behav 26:2891–2896

HIV and migrants – Monitoring the implementation of the Dublin Declaration on partnership to fight HIV/AIDS in Europe and Central Asia: 2022 progress report [web site] (2023) (https://www.ecdc.europa.eu/en/publications-data/hiv-and-migrants-monitoring-implementation-dublin-declaration-partnership-fight, Accessed 10 Dec 2024)

Implementing the global health sector strategies on HIV, viral hepatitis and sexually transmitted infections, 2022–2030: report on progress and gaps 2024 [web site] (https://www.who.int/publications/i/item/9789240094925, Accessed 10 Dec 2024)

Irons R (2022) Aquí viene una Veneca más': Venezuelan migrants and 'the sexual question' in Peru. Anthropol Med 29:323–337

Jordan K, Lewis TP, Roberts B (2021) Quality in crisis: a systematic review of the quality of health systems in humanitarian settings. Confl Heal 15:7

Kamenshchikova A, Peters CMM, Nöstlinger C, Rice B, Ford N, Ravasi G et al (2024) Interventions to ensure access to and continuity of HIV care for international migrants: an evidence synthesis. Lancet HIV 11:e873–e884

Korenromp EL, Sabin K, Stover J, Brown T, Johnson LF, Martin-Hughes R et al (2024) New HIV infections among key populations and their partners in 2010 and 2022, by world region: a multisources estimation. JAIDS J Acquir Immune Defic Syndr 95:e34

Kularatne R, Blondeel K, Kasaro M, Maseko V, Bosomprah S, Silva R et al (2024) Clinic-based evaluation of point-of-care dual HIV/syphilis rapid diagnostic tests at primary healthcare antenatal facilities in South Africa and Zambia. BMC Infect Dis 24:600

Kumar A, Parihar A, Panda U, Parihar DS (2022) Microfluidics-based point-of-care testing (POCT) devices in dealing with waves of COVID-19 pandemic: the emerging solution. ACS Appl Bio Mater 5:2046–2068

Lebano A, Hamed S, Bradby H, Gil-Salmerón A, Durá-Ferrandis E, Garcés-Ferrer J et al (2020) Migrants' and refugees' health status and healthcare in Europe: a scoping literature review. BMC Public Health 20:1039

Liu M-L, Xia Y, Wu X-Z, Huang J-Q, Guo X-G (2017) Loop-mediated isothermal amplification of Neisseria gonorrhoeae porA pseudogene: a rapid and reliable method to detect gonorrhea. AMB Express 7:48

Liu A, Coleman K, Bojan K, Serrano PA, Oyedele T, Garcia A et al (2019) Developing a mobile app (LYNX) to support linkage to HIV/sexually transmitted infection testing and pre-exposure prophylaxis for young men who have sex with men: protocol for a randomized controlled trial. JMIR Res Protoc 8:e10659

Manabe YC (2023) The impact of COVID-19 pandemic on technologic and process innovation in point-of-care diagnostics for sexually transmitted infections. Clin Biochem 117:75–83

Mann S, Mougammadou Z, Wohlfahrt J, Elmahdi R (2024) Post-migration HIV acquisition: a systematic review and meta-analysis. Epidemiol Infect 152:e49

Migration, Human Mobility and HIV [web site] (https://www.iom.int/resources/migration-human-mobility-and-hiv, Accessed 10 Dec 2024)

Mitjà O, Padovese V, Folch C, Rossoni I, Marks M, Arias MAR et al (2023) Epidemiology and determinants of reemerging bacterial sexually transmitted infections (STIs) and emerging STIs in Europe. Lancet Reg Health–Eur 34. https://doi.org/10.1016/j.lanepe.2023.100742

Monitoring HIV pre-exposure prophylaxis programmes in the EU/EEA [web site] (2022) (https://www.ecdc.europa.eu/en/publications-data/monitoring-hiv-pre-exposure-prophylaxis-programmes-eueea, Accessed 10 Dec 2024)

Mosler Vidal E, Laczko F, International Organization for Migration (eds) (2022) Migration and the SDGs: measuring progress: an edited volume. International Organization for Migration, Geneva, Switzerland

New York Declaration for Refugees and Migrants [web site] (https://www.unhcr.org/media/new-york-declaration-refugees-and-migrants-0, Accessed 17 Dec 2024)

Padovese V, Farrugia A, Almabrok Ali Ghath S, Rossoni I (2021) Sexually transmitted infections' epidemiology and knowledge, attitude and practice survey in a set of migrants attending the sexual health clinic in Malta. J Eur Acad Dermatol Venereol 35:509–516

Panchenko S, Gabster A, Mayaud P, Erausquin JT (2024) Sexual health challenges in migrant, immigrant, and displaced populations 2022–2023. Curr Opin Infect Dis 37:46

Point-of-care tests for sexually transmitted infections: target product profiles [web site] (https://www.who.int/publications/i/item/9789240077102, Accessed 18 Dec 2024)

Poljak M, Cuschieri K, Waheed D-E-N, Baay M, Vorsters A (2021) Impact of the COVID-19 pandemic on human papillomavirus-based testing services to support cervical cancer screening. Acta Dermatovenerol Alp Pannonica Adriat 30:21–26

Prequalified In Vitro Diagnostics | WHO – Prequalification of Medical Products (IVDs, Medicines, Vaccines and Immunization Devices, Vector Control) [web site] (https://extranet.who.int/prequal/vitro-diagnostics/prequalified-vitro-diagnostics, Accessed 13 Mar 2025)

Rodriguez NM, Wong WS, Liu L, Dewar R, Klapperich CM (2016) A fully integrated paperfluidic molecular diagnostic chip for the extraction, amplification, and detection of nucleic acids from clinical samples. Lab Chip 16:753–763

Rodriguez-Mateos P, Ngamsom B, Ameyo D, Wakaba P, Shiluli C, Iles A et al (2023) Integrated microscale immiscible phase extraction and isothermal amplification for colorimetric detection of Neisseria gonorrhoeae. Anal Bioanal Chem 415:5129–5137

Santoso D, Asfia SKBM, Mello MB, Baggaley RC, Johnson CC, Chow EPF et al (2022) HIV prevalence ratio of international migrants compared to their native-born counterparts: a systematic review and meta-analysis. EClinicalMedicine 53. https://doi.org/10.1016/j.eclinm.2022.101661

Sexually transmitted infections (STIs) [web site] (https://www.who.int/news-room/fact-sheets/detail/sexually-transmitted-infections-(stis), Accessed 10 Dec 2024)

Shephard M, Matthews S, Kularatne R, Andrewartha K, Blondeel K, Alvarez C et al (2024a) Independent clinic-based evaluation of point-of-care testing for the screening of Chlamydia trachomatis, Neisseria gonorrhoea and Trichomonas vaginalis in women-at-risk in Australia, Guatemala, Morocco, and South Africa. BMC Infect Dis 24:277

Shephard M, Matthews S, Andrewartha K, Dimech W, Cabuang L, Barbara C et al (2024b) Quality control and external quality assessment for the independent clinic-based evaluation of point-of-care testing to detect Chlamydia trachomatis, Neisseria gonorrhoeae and Trichomonas vaginalis in eight countries. BMC Infect Dis 24:203

Sherriff N, Mirandola M, Silva R, Cordioli M, Sawyer A, Gios L et al (2024) Independent clinic-based evaluation of dual POCTs for screening for HIV and syphilis in men who have sex with men in Italy, Malta, Peru, and the United Kingdom. BMC Infect Dis 24:192

Soe NN, Latt PM, King A, Lee D, Phillips TR, Fairley CK et al (2025) What do people want from an AI-assisted screening app for sexually transmitted infection-related anogenital lesions: a discrete choice experiment. The Patient 18:131–143

Sweileh WM (2024) Analysis and mapping of global research publications on point-of-care testing for infectious diseases. J Eval Clin Pract 30:945–953

Tanner NA, Zhang Y, Evans TC Jr (2015) Visual detection of isothermal nucleic acid amplification using pH-sensitive dyes. BioTechniques 58:59–68

Tayyab M, Barrett D, Van Riel G, Liu S, Reinius B, Scharfe C et al (2023) Digital assay for rapid electronic quantification of clinical pathogens using DNA nanoballs. Sci Adv 9:eadi4997

The diagnostics landscape for sexually transmitted infections [web site] (https://www.who.int/publications/i/item/9789240077126, Accessed 18 Dec 2024)

The diagnostics landscape for sexually transmitted infections [web site] (https://www.who.int/publications/i/item/9789240077126, Accessed 13 Mar 2025)

Toskin I, Murtagh M, Peeling RW, Blondeel K, Cordero J, Kiarie J (2017a) Advancing prevention of sexually transmitted infections through point-of-care testing: target product profiles and landscape analysis. Sex Transm Infect 93:S69–S80

Toskin I, Blondeel K, Peeling RW, Deal C, Kiarie J (2017b) Advancing point of care diagnostics for the control and prevention of STIs: the way forward. Sex Transm Infect 93:S81–S88

Townsend H, Hobbs J, Kaylor S, Cody S, Callihan M (2024) Point-of-care STI testing in rural settings: a feasibility project. Public Health Nurs 41:1202–1205

Tsorou C, Williams A, van den Boogaard W, Staderini N, Repetto E, Terzidis A et al (2024) Point-of-care diagnostics for sexually transmitted infections among migrants in Greece. Public Health Action 14:14–19

Taylor D, Lunny C, Wong T, Gilbert M, Li N, Lester R, Krajden M, Hoang L, Ogilvie G (2013) Self-collected versus clinician-collected sampling for sexually transmitted infections: a systematic review and meta-analysis protocol. Syst Rev 10;2:93. https://doi.org/10.1186/2046-4053-2-93. PMID: 24112441; PMCID: PMC3851982

Vargas S, Calvo G, Qquellon J, Vasquez F, Blondeel K, Ballard R et al (2022) Point-of-care testing for sexually transmitted infections in low-resource settings. Clin Microbiol Infect 28:946–951

Vasylyeva TI, Horyniak D, Bojorquez I, Pham MD (2022) Left behind on the path to 90-90-90: understanding and responding to HIV among displaced people. J Int AIDS Soc 25:e26031

Venter W, Coleman J, Chan VL, Shubber Z, Phatsoane M, Gorgens M et al (2018) Improving linkage to HIV care through mobile phone apps: randomized controlled trial. JMIR Mhealth Uhealth 6:e155

Wong A, Applegate T, Boettiger DC, Varma R, Guy R, Medland N (2024) Unnecessary antibiotic use in men who have sex with men (MSM) with anogenital symptoms attending a sexual health clinic: a retrospective analysis. Sex Transm Infect 100:435–441

World Health Organization (2022) Global health sector strategies on, respectively, HIV, viral hepatitis and sexually transmitted infections for the period 2022–2030, 1st edn. World Health Organization, Geneva

World Health Organization (2023) Laboratory and point-of-care diagnostic testing for sexually transmitted infections, including HIV, 1st edn. World Health Organization, Geneva

World Health Organization (2024) Target product profiles for human papillomavirus screening tests to detect cervical pre-cancer and cancer. World Health Organization. (https://iris.who.int/handle/10665/379099, Accessed 4 Dec 2024)

Yang Z, Wang J, Qi Y, Shi Y, Li F, Wang W et al (2024) A novel detection method based on MIRA-CRISPR/Cas13a-LFD targeting the repeated DNA sequence of Trichomonas vaginalis. Parasit Vectors 17:14

Zhang Y, Zhang P, Chen L, Kaushik A, Hu K, Wang T-H (2020) ddRFC: a scalable multiplexed droplet digital nucleic acid amplification test platform. Biosens Bioelectron 167:112499

Zhang J, Su Z, Luo Q, Wei H, Liao J, Chen W et al (2025) *Ttr*Ago-mediated nucleic acid detection system and portable device for rapid detection of sexually transmitted diseases. Biosens Bioelectron 272:117029

Zhou H, Cai Y, He L, Li T, Wang Z, Li L et al (2025) Phase transition of wax enabling CRISPR diagnostics for automatic at-home testing of multiple sexually transmitted infection pathogens. Small Weinh Bergstr Ger 21:e2407931

Conclusions: Towards Integrated, Rights-Based, Interdisciplinary and Inter-Sectoral Frameworks for Migrant Health and Well-Being

11

Isotta Rossoni and Valeska Padovese

Contents

Abstract

On World Health Day 2025, the United Nations Network on Migration made a powerful statement in support of migrants, underscoring that they "are not merely recipients of healthcare; they are frontline workers, caregivers and key contributors to resilient health systems and community well-being", and ensuring their access to health "strengthens societies, reduces public health costs and fosters more inclusive, sustainable communities" (United Nations Network on Migration 2025). This book highlights the vital role of migrants and refugees and advances for an interdisciplinary, rights-based approach to sexual and reproductive health (SRH). Traditional practices like disease screening, vaccination, and family planning are important but insufficient to address migrants' complex needs or to promote a holistic understanding of sexual well-being (Singer and Clair 2003; Tsai and Burns 2015).

On World Health Day 2025, the United Nations Network on Migration made a powerful statement in support of migrants, underscoring that they "are not merely recipients of healthcare; they are frontline workers, caregivers and key contributors to resilient health systems and community well-being", and ensuring their access to health "strengthens societies, reduces public health costs and fosters more inclusive, sustainable communities" (United Nations Network on Migration 2025). This book highlights the vital role of migrants and refugees and advances for an interdisciplinary, rights-based approach to sexual and reproductive health (SRH). Traditional practices like disease screening, vaccination, and family planning are important but insufficient to address migrants' complex needs or to promote a holistic understanding of sexual well-being (Singer and Clair 2003; Tsai and Burns 2015).

I. Rossoni (✉)
Van Vollenhoven Institute -Leiden Law School, Leiden University, Leiden, The Netherlands

V. Padovese
Genitourinary Clinic, Department of Dermatology and Venereology, Mater Dei Hospital, Msida, Malta
e-mail: valeska.padovese@gov.mt

V. Padovese, I. Rossoni (eds.), *Intersections of Sexual Health, Migration and Sexualised Violence*, Sustainable Development Goals Series, https://doi.org/10.1007/978-3-032-20707-4_11

Research shows that migrants and displaced people face multiple, overlapping vulnerabilities (Singer and Clair 2003) that affect their health beyond single conditions. Structural, institutional, community, and interpersonal factors all limit access to sexual and reproductive health (SRH) (Logie et al. 2024). Crucially, migration itself is a key social determinant of health. Legal status, living and working conditions, transit and reception contexts—including closed detention—and migration trajectories contribute to health-related risks (World Health Organization Regional Office for the Eastern Mediterranean 2021). Effective policies should address not only biomedical needs but also the broader social, legal, and migration systems that create vulnerability.

Syndemics theory emphasizes how multiple epidemics or health issues co-occur, interact synergistically, and are driven by common social and structural determinants (Singer and Clair 2003; Singer 2009). For migrant populations, this means that sexual health risks often overlap with migration-related vulnerabilities, mental health burdens, gender-based violence, and socioeconomic exclusion. Syndemic and human-rights approaches argue that determinants such as legal status, housing, employment, and discrimination must be tackled if we are to curtail the clustering of risks (Mezzina et al. 2022). There is a dire need for integrated interventions that recognize and promptly respond to the interplay of sexual health, violence prevention, mental health, migration justice, and broader social policy. This comprehensive approach acknowledges that health outcomes for migrants are shaped by interconnected determinants and calls for policies and practices that bridge these domains, fostering collaboration across sectors such as healthcare, legal advocacy, housing, employment, and education. By building partnerships between governmental agencies, community organizations, and affected populations, solutions can be designed that address root causes and adapt to the lived realities of migrants and refugees. Such synergy not only strengthens health and well-being but also advances equity, resilience, and social cohesion within increasingly diverse societies.

Linked to this is the imperative to adopt a sexual well-being orientation rather than simply a disease-control approach. As some scholars have recently argued, sexual well-being is a distinct concept that builds on sexual health, adding the dimensions of pleasure, autonomy, intimacy, rights, and equity. It shifts the narrative from "what disease or risk can we prevent?" to "what does it mean for someone to have fulfilling, safe, pleasurable, respectful sexual lives?"(Mitchell et al. 2021). This collection urges us to complement this reflection with an additional question: "how can the vulnerabilities and risks that prevent individuals from having fulfilling, safe, pleasurable, respectful sexual lives in the context of migration and displacement, be reduced?". While the World Health Organization definition of sexual health already emphasizes a respectful and positive approach, the implementation of health-based interventions in practice remains strongly risk-oriented (World Health Organization 2022). Integrating sexual well-being with an emphasis on rights, non-discrimination, and violence prevention ought to be a key priority of SRH policies for migrants.

Within this wider approach, comprehensive sexuality education (CSE) emerges as a key pillar. Migrants and refugees—especially young people, those out of formal schooling, women, LGBTIQA+ individuals and those with irregular status—are often excluded from standard CSE and sexual health services because of cultural, linguistic, legal, and mobility barriers. Focus-group research with migrants across European countries shows strong demand for sexual health education that is culturally responsive, uses native or simplified languages, addresses safer sex practices, anatomy, consent, and relationships, and integrates socio-cultural sensitivities (Konstantinou et al. 2025). Globally, systematic reviews show that CSE in humanitarian and LMIC settings can reduce risky sexual behaviours and improve SRH outcomes (Desrosiers et al. 2020). Yet in migration contexts, educational access, cultural relevance, and connectivity to services remain under-addressed (Kirby and Laris 2009). While cultural adaptation is sorely needed, educators in various LMICs identify tensions when implementing CSE due to cultural and religious resistance, unclear roles, and content mismatches (Shibuya et al. 2023). In light of this, more research should focus on culturally appropriate CSE in view of embedding it in sexual health policy and educational interventions for migrants, which are rooted in their lived experiences and rely on their active contribution.

While this collection does not address the issue of masculinity(ies), the role of CSE in engaging men and boys cannot be overlooked. Even if sexual and gender-based violence (SGBV) has long been recognized as a central concern in migrant health, prevention strategies continue to focus predominantly on women as victims, with limited attention being devoted to men and masculinities. Yet research across humanitarian and migration settings demonstrates that rigid gender norms, patriarchal expectations, and disrupted social roles during displacement can contribute both to men's perpetration of violence and to their own experiences of sexual victimization (United Nations Entity for Gender Equality and the Empowerment of Women (UN Women) 2023; Reidy et al. 2022). Moreover, men's and boys' beliefs around sex, sexuality, and sexual health can impede women's access to SRH services, including in cases of violence (Brennan-Wilson et al. 2024). Addressing masculinities is therefore essential to violence prevention and to promoting sexual well-being. Interventions that engage men as allies in gender equality, encourage reflection on masculinity and power, and integrate discussions of consent, emotional regulation and non-violence have shown promise in both low- and high-income settings (Gordon et al. 2012; Jewkes et al. 2015). Incorporating such approaches into migrant and refugee programmes can reduce violence, improve couple communication and support broader well-being. Critically, this work must include men without displacing women's voices, situating masculinity transformation within wider gender-justice agendas.

From a policy and intervention perspective, several interlinked imperatives emerge. Legal frameworks must guarantee access for all migrants, regardless of status, to SRH services including contraception, safe abortion, STI/HIV prevention and care, psychosocial support, and gender-based violence prevention. Health policies should be combined with dignified migration, labour, education, and social protection. It is crucial for reception centres, housing programmes, employment regulation, legal aid, and integration services to embed SRH and sexual well-being pathways. Relatedly, data and monitoring systems must be disaggregated by migration status, gender, sexual orientation, and migration pathway and include indicators for sexual well-being, violence, and psychosexual care, not just disease metrics. Funding and resource allocation should prioritize these intersectional approaches rather than disease-specific silos. Crucially, migrant voices, communities of origin and destination, LGBTIQA+ migrants, sex-worker migrants, and those with lived experience should be engaged as equal partners in policy and programme design, implementation, and evaluation. It is evident that a transformative shift is necessary—one that reimagines sexual and reproductive health not as an isolated medical concern but as an integral part of social justice and community resilience. This requires dismantling barriers at every level, from restrictive legal policies and inadequate funding to cultural stigma and the marginalization of migrant voices in policy discussions. By situating migrants and refugees as active agents in shaping their own health trajectories and ensuring that care systems are accessible, intersectional, and attuned to lived experience, we pave the way for more equitable and sustainable outcomes. Policymakers, practitioners, and researchers must collaborate to embed these principles into practice, ensuring that the rights, dignity, and well-being of all migrants are upheld as central to public health advancement.

Finally, we must reflect on the broader global justice and historical context. Migration flows are often shaped by structural injustices—conflict, climate change, colonial legacies, and economic exclusion—that continue to drive inequities in health, sexuality, and rights. The syndemic lens reminds us that clustering of health burdens and social vulnerabilities is not accidental but socially produced. For migrants, sexual health vulnerabilities are shaped by the intersecting inequalities of gender, race, coloniality, legal status and global power. Our policy frameworks therefore must not only aim for service delivery but also challenge discrimination, reform migration regimes that produce legal precarity, and ensure labour rights and equitable access to social protection and education. Sexual and reproductive health for migrants becomes, therefore, a matter of human rights and social justice, not simply technical service provision.

To advance sexual and reproductive health, violence prevention and sexual well-being for migrants and refugees globally, we must move from fragmented, risk-based responses to integrated, rights-based, interdisciplinary, and intersectoral frameworks. Sexual well-being, culturally appropriate education, structural reform, community-led interventions, and data that reflect complexity must be the pillars of policy change. Only by aligning SRH with migration, socio-economic, education, and legal systems can we truly hope to leave no one behind.

References

Brennan-Wilson A, Marques M, Coates A, Amin A, Garry J, Tomlinson M, Nyembezi A, George A, Lohan M (2024) Masculinities and sexual and reproductive health and rights: a global research priority setting exercise. Lancet Glob Health 12(5):e882–e890. https://doi.org/10.1016/S2214-109X(24)00053-6

Desrosiers A, Betancourt T, Kergoat Y et al (2020) A systematic review of sexual and reproductive health interventions for young people in humanitarian and lower- and middle-income country settings. BMC Public Health 20:666. https://doi.org/10.1186/s12889-020-08818-y

Gordon DM, Hunter B, Woods LN, Tinney B, Bostic B, Malone S et al (2012) Increasing outreach, connection, and services to low-income non-custodial fathers: how did we get here and what do we know. Fathering 10(1):101–111. https://doi.org/10.3149/fth.1001.101. PMID: 24817832; PMCID: PMC4015970

Jewkes R, Flood M, Lang J (2015) From work with men and boys to changes of social norms and reduction of inequities in gender relations: a conceptual shift in prevention of violence against women and girls. Lancet 385(9977):1580–1589. https://doi.org/10.1016/S0140-6736(14)61683-4

Kirby D, Laris BA (2009) The impact of sex and HIV education programs in schools and communities: a review of program evaluations. The World Bank

Konstantinou E, Murto T, Bacatum C et al (2025) Migrants' perceptions and needs in sexual health education: a focus group study. Sex Cult 29:943–962. https://doi.org/10.1007/s12119-024-10307-y

Logie CH, MacKenzie F, Malama K, Lorimer N, Lad A, Zhao M et al (2024) Sexual and reproductive health among forcibly displaced persons in urban environments in low and middle-income countries: scoping review findings. Reprod Health 21:51. https://doi.org/10.1186/s12978-024-01780-7

Mezzina R, Gopikumar V, Jenkins J, Saraceno B, Sashidharan SP (2022) Social vulnerability and mental health inequalities in the "syndemic": call for action. Front Psych 13:894370. https://doi.org/10.3389/fpsyt.2022.894370. PMID: 35747101; PMCID: PMC9210067

Mitchell KR, Lewis R, O'Sullivan LF, Fortenberry JD (2021) What is sexual wellbeing, and why does it matter for public health? Lancet Public Health 6(8):e608–e613. https://doi.org/10.1016/S2468-2667(21)00099-2

Reidy DE, Leone RM, Bogen KW, Swahn MH (2022) Chapter 6 - The culture of masculinity and sexual violence: raising boys to be nonviolent men. In: Engaging boys and men in sexual assault prevention. Elsevier Inc, pp 125–148

Shibuya F, Estrada CA, Sari DP et al (2023) Teachers' conflicts in implementing comprehensive sexuality education: a qualitative systematic review and meta-synthesis. Trop Med Health 51:18. https://doi.org/10.1186/s41182-023-00508-w

Singer M (2009) Introduction to Syndemics: a critical systems approach to public and community health, 1st edn. Jossey-Bass, San Francisco

Singer M, Clair S (2003) Syndemics and public health: reconceptualizing disease in bio-social context. Med Anthropol Q 17(4):423–441

Tsai AC, Burns BFO (2015) Syndemics of psychosocial problems and HIV risk: a systematic review of empirical tests of the disease interaction concept. Soc Sci Med 139:26–35

United Nations Entity for Gender Equality and the Empowerment of Women (UN Women) (2023) Men, masculinities and humanitarian settings: a mapping of the state of research and practice-based evidence. UN Women, New York. [cited 2025 Oct 24]. Available from: https://knowledge.unwomen.org/sites/default/files/2023-08/men-masculinities-and-humanitarian-settings-en.pdf

United Nations Network on Migration (2025) United Nations network on migration statement for world health day 2025. UN Network on Migration, Geneva. [cited 2025 Oct 24]. Available from: https://migrationnetwork.un.org/statements/united-nations-network-migration-statement-world-health-day-2025

World Health Organization (2022) Redefining sexual health for benefits throughout life. WHO, Geneva. Available from: https://www.who.int/news/item/11-02-2022-redefining-sexual-health-for-benefits--throughout-life

World Health Organization Regional Office for the Eastern Mediterranean (2021) The social and structural determinants of sexual and reproductive health and rights in migrants and refugees: a systematic review of reviews. East Mediterr Health J 27(12):1203–1213

Correction to: Caring for Refugees and Migrants: Volunteer and Professional Aid Workers

Anne Jachmann and Katharina Wahedi

Correction to:
Chapter 9 in: V. Padovese, I. Rossoni (eds.), *Intersections of Sexual Health, Migration and Sexualised Violence*, Sustainable Development Goals Series, https://doi.org/10.1007/978-3-032-20707-4_9

This original version of Chapter 9 has been updated with revised Figures 9.1 and 9.3.

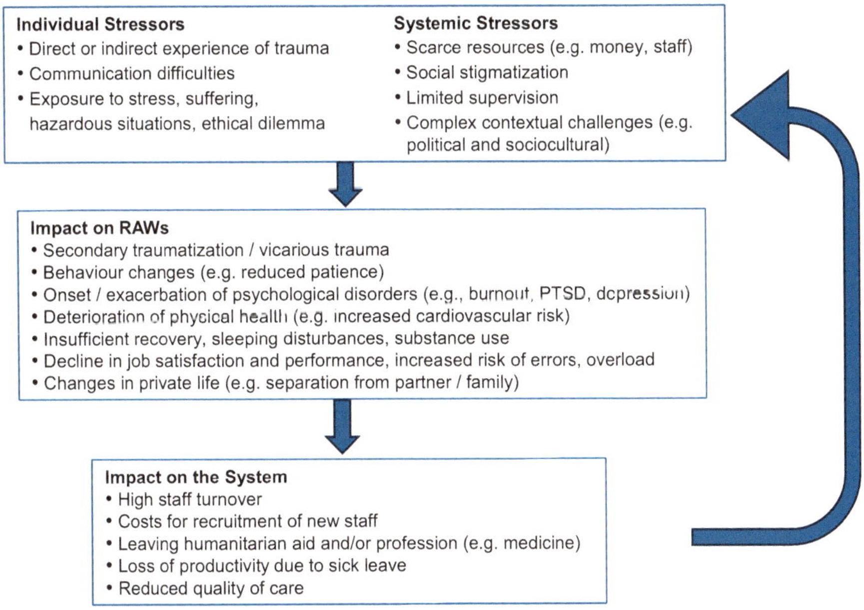

Fig. 9.1 Working in the field of MRH: exposure to stressors and their potential negative impacts. Adapted from Jachmann et al. 2024

The updated version of this chapter can be found at
https://doi.org/10.1007/978-3-032-20707-4_9

V. Padovese, I. Rossoni (eds.), *Intersections of Sexual Health, Migration and Sexualised Violence*, Sustainable Development Goals Series, https://doi.org/10.1007/978-3-032-20707-4_12

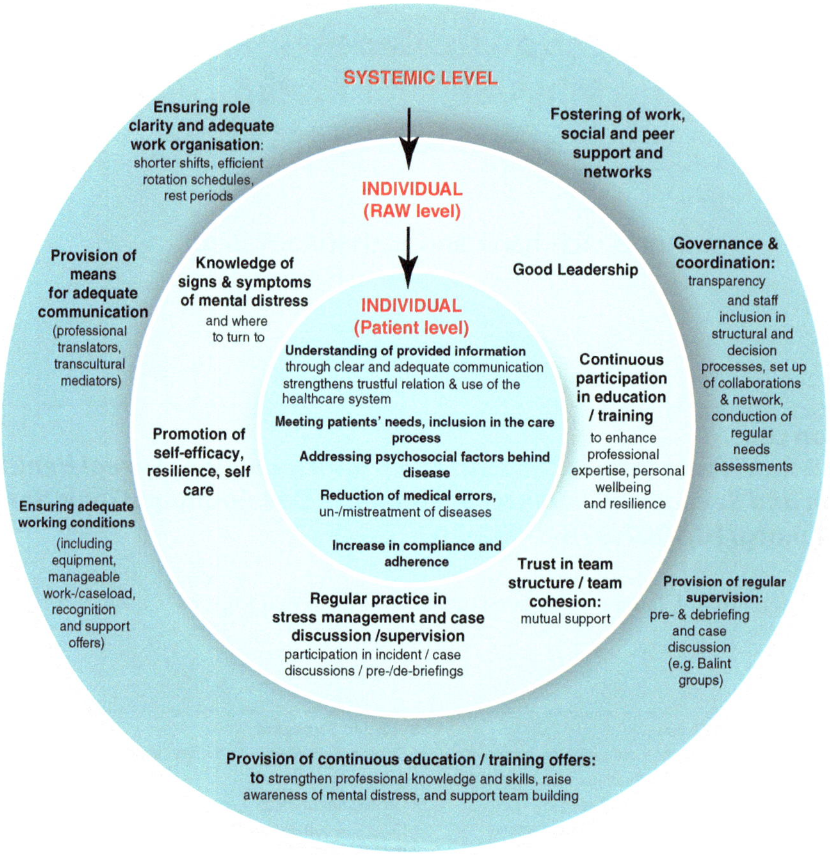

Fig. 9.3 Protective factors and their consequences within MRH work. Adapted from Jachmann et al. 2024 and Jachmann et al. 2025

Batch number: 10615152

Printed by Printforce, the Netherlands